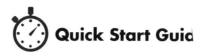 **Quick Start Guide**

The
ALKALINE DIET
SOLUTION

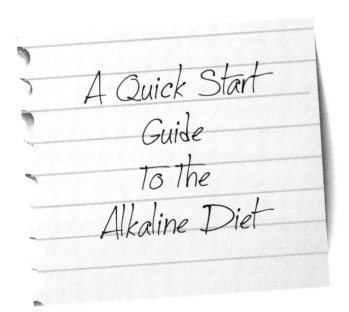

A Quick Start Guide To The Alkaline Diet

Lose Weight, Improve Your Health and Feel Great!

Plus over 90 Alkaline Friendly Recipes

First published in 2015 by Erin Rose Publishing

Text and illustration copyright © 2015 Erin Rose Publishing

Design: Julie Anson

ISBN: 978-0-9928232-9-0

A CIP record for this book is available from the British Library.

DISCLAIMER: This book is for informational purposes only and not intended as a substitute for the medical advice, diagnosis or treatment of a physician or qualified healthcare provider. The reader should consult a physician before undertaking a new health care regimen and in all matters relating to his/her health, and particularly with respect to any symptoms that may require diagnosis or medical attention.

Whilst every care has been taken in compiling the recipes for this book we cannot accept responsibility for any problems which arise as a result of preparing one of the recipes. The author and publisher disclaim responsibility for any adverse effects that may arise from the use or application of the recipes in this book. Some of the recipes in this book include nuts and eggs. If you have an egg or nut allergy it's important to avoid these. It is recommended that children, pregnant women, the elderly or anyone who has an immune system disorder avoid eating raw eggs.

CONTENTS

Recipes

INTRODUCTION

"Not another fad diet where you lose 5 lbs in a week and put it all back on again!"

Let's face it, that's what many of us think when we hear about another celebrity endorsed diet craze and it's often true! We know that yo-yo dieting is bad for us but often we lurch from one diet to another trying to lose weight and more importantly trying to get healthier. We already know the most effective and healthiest way to lose weight is by making healthy adjustments to our everyday diet that are sensible, sustainable and good for our health, both in the short and long term. But with so much conflicting information out there, how do we know what a healthy diet is?

It's agreed that fruit and vegetables are good for us but the quantities are often too low in proportion to the rest of our meals. However, on the alkaline diet it's different. By making some key changes you can really improve your well-being and lose weight. In this book we give you a 7 day alkaline menu plan to help your body cleanse and detoxify, plus you'll discover how to take a fresh approach to healthy eating and be able to achieve natural weight loss by making sensible changes to your diet without being obsessed. You really can achieve great results and attain better health, weight and vitality. You won't look back.

In this Quick Start Guide we'll tell you how to get started alkalising your diet. This book gives you the essential information without the jargon. It provides you with the key principles, comprehensive yet detailed food lists with plenty of useful tips together with ample recipes which are simple, easy and delicious. Importantly, the recipes use everyday ingredients because we know how difficult it can be finding obscure foods. It's simply whole-foods and clean eating! The sooner you start the sooner you see results. Are you ready?

What Is the Alkaline Diet?

The alkaline diet is not new. It's been a useful, holistic approach to treating many illnesses for decades however it's now gaining credibility and publicity because it's an effective antidote to our modern fast-food diets and stressed digestive systems which are taking their toll resulting with rising obesity, chronic illnesses and immune problems.

Following a diet consisting of mostly alkaline-forming foods is a powerful way to neutralise harmful excess acids in your body, bringing about positive changes to your health. Alkalining enables you to balance the pH levels of your body and you'll be able to monitor how effective this is, not only by how good you feel but you can even test your own pH levels.

The benefits of alkalining are far reaching. By reducing the acids in your body and encouraging your body to cleanse of toxins which have built up, you can see and feel the improvements in a fairly short time. Many people report improvements beyond their healthy weight loss, with them feeling more alert and focused, plus their complexion and skin tone is clearer.

A diet which is high in acid-forming foods like red meat, bread, cakes, sugar and caffeine can have a detrimental effect on the body and unfortunately what we class as a 'normal diet' is full of these ingredients which create excess acidity. Over-acidity prevents the body from functioning at an optimum level and can make it difficult to eliminate toxins. Our bodies then struggle to heal fully so illnesses build up and lead to worsening health. When the body is too acidic, the lungs and kidneys struggle to keep the pH balance at a healthy level. The results of excess acidity aren't good and they have been linked with a wide range of health problems from muscle and joint problems to fertility issues and chronic diseases. It can't all be blamed on diet. An unhealthy and stressful lifestyle is also a factor but a good diet is essential to counteract it.

The goal is to maintain a healthy equilibrium to make things easier for your body by eating a diet of mainly alkaline foods.

Despite the foods own pH level, it will have either an alkaline-forming or acid-forming affect on the body. It's not the pH level of the food itself which is the problem but what it does do the body when digested. For instance lemons which taste and are acidic actually have a strongly alkalising affect on the body.

The affects of excess acidity in the body have been linked with the following health problems:

- Allergies
- Bloating
- Cardiovascular Disease
- Cancer
- Constipation
- Chronic Fatigue
- Diabetes
- Fertility issues
- Irritable Bowel Syndrome
- Inflammatory illnesses, joint and muscle problems
- Low immunity causing frequent colds
- Lack of concentration
- Poor energy
- Skin problems
- Weight problems, such as inability to lose weight

NB: Check with your doctor that it's safe for you to make dietary changes, especially if you have any health issues.

So now that we've got the negatives out of the way, let's be upbeat about this. The good news is the effects of excess acidity in the body are reversible!

Alkalising your diet combats over-acidity.

By reducing your intake of acid forming foods such as sugar, caffeine, alcohol and junk food and supplementing it with strongly alkaline-forming foods such as green vegetables like spinach, kale and broccoli and swapping to more plant based protein, you can achieve a healthier acid-alkaline balance in your body.

Your digestive system is your body's power house for extracting nutrients and providing optimum nourishment to keep us in peak health. But overload your digestion and it will struggle, like adding too much fuel to a fire when the flame is already dwindling. It needs taking care of without being overwhelmed. Eating more alkaline-forming foods takes a load off your digestion, helps reduce the signs of premature ageing, boosts your metabolism and rewards you with extra vigour and vitality. By making healthy changes you are safe-guarding your future well-being and prevention is always better than cure.

To achieve this, increase the alkaline portion of your meals to approximately 80% and have only 20% of acid-forming food. So visualise that in your mind. Just over ¾ of your plate should consist of alkaline, plant-based foods and in particular green leafy vegetables.

Team that with some simple key principles and you can change your diet and health for the better. It really can be that simple!

The Principles Of The Alkaline Diet

If you are thinking this all sounds rather daunting, feel reassured that there are only a few key points that you need to remember to implement a more alkaline diet. Here they are!

The Principles

- Eat at least 80% alkaline foods at every meal.
- Don't eat meals consisting of solely acid-forming foods.
- If you are particularly acidic you can further reduce your intake of acid-forming foods.
- If you wish to eat just alkalising foods, do so for no more than 1-2 weeks.

Your goal is to reduce the acid-forming foods and increase the alkaline-forming foods. When we've been advised to eat a healthy balanced diet in the past we often don't really know what that means. Typically our meals focus on the protein element and the majority of our plates are stacked with carbohydrates, but it's about shifting this so that vegetables and plant-based foods are in the greatest quantity.

For some, eating more alkaline-forming foods will require a complete overhaul of their diet, for others it's less dramatic and mostly requires a shift in the ratio of protein, vegetables and carbohydrates. Making changes to the amount of alkaline foods you consume lightens the load on your digestive system which makes if more efficient and therefore able to process what you're putting in. It also takes the strain off the liver and kidneys. The way food is cooked can also change how it affects your body. For instance potatoes are naturally alkaline- forming however once they are deep-fried in oil they become acidifying.

You can monitor your pH levels to give you an indication of the internal environment of your body based on your body fluids, even though the pH values of different parts of the body are different. This can not only encourage and motivate you but can help you to decide if you need to make any adjustments to your alkaline food intake. In other words, if you are particularly acidic you may wish to further decrease your acid-forming food intake.

The pH value, used to determine how acid/alkaline something is, falls across a spectrum from 1-14. In that range 0 is the most acidic, 14 is the most alkaline and right in the middle at 7 is neutral or basic.

The body is more alkaline and pH readings of between 7.3 and 7.5 are the most compatible with health. Normal bodily functions happen between these levels. Urinary pH of 7.4, which is slightly alkaline, is considered good whereas if you are testing your saliva, aim for between 6.5 and 7.0. You don't have to monitor your progress using the strips but some people find it gives them motivation and encourages them when they see results.

You can test the pH level of your urine or saliva at home. To do this test you will need litmus strips which are available from pharmacies or you can order them online. Checking the pH level of your urine will indicate how acidic your internal environment is. Also note that dehydration, caffeine, alcohol and some medication change your acidity levels.

How To Get Started

First, pick the right time. If you have an upcoming wedding or birthday party you may be thinking you don't want to start on the alkaline diet just yet OR you may decide that an upcoming social event **is** the perfect motivation you need to feel good, lose a few excess pounds and put a spring in your step.

Familiarise yourself with the food lists so that they become second nature and you can steer clear of highly acidifying foods. It's not always possible to avoid them entirely and we want you to enjoy what you eat without obsessing over what you can and can't eat. Think about what you want to achieve and set your goal. For some of you a normal diet will consist of a great deal of fast/junk food so implementing vast changes are going to seem extreme. You may prefer to cut back on as much of the acidic food as you can. Once you've gotten into a routine and your taste buds have adjusted to new subtler flavours you can improve things further if you wish and it won't seem too radical.

You can embark on the 7 day detox and really kick start your alkaline regime by cleansing your body and you'll see the benefits very quickly indeed. The 7 day detox is more restrictive although it is only for a short while.

So, if you'd rather increase your intake of alkaline foods gradually you can do this just by bearing in mind the 80/20 principle. You may find it easier to stick to if you break yourself in gently. Following the 80/20 principle on a daily basis is sustainable and will also bring about great results.

The choice is yours – 7 day detox to begin with or straight to everyday alkalining? However, if your health is below par and your pH levels are very acidic, it's best to allow you body to heal and detoxify by removing even weakly-acidifying foods temporarily.

Acid-Forming Foods List

This is a list of acid-forming foods so **REDUCE** or **AVOID** these.

Grains/Starches:

- Wheat and wheat containing products such as bread, cereals, pasta, couscous, cakes and biscuits.

Dairy:

- Cow's milk dairy produce; milk, butter, cream, cheese and ice cream

- Ghee

Proteins:

- Beef

- Chicken

- Lamb

- Pork

- Turkey

- Fish

- Shellfish

Drinks:

- Alcohol

- Fizzy drinks

- Carbonated Water

- Coffee

- Cola

- Concentrated fruit juices

- Energy drinks

- Soda water

- Tea

- Tonic water

Sweeteners:

- Sugar and products containing sugar: jams, spreads, sweets, fizzy drinks, chocolate, ready-made sauces, dressings and marinades containing sugar.

- Artificial sweeteners

- Fructose

- High fructose corn syrup

Weakly Acidifying Foods

This is a list of weakly acid-forming foods which provide essential nutrients to the body and can be eaten when combined with more alkaline foods.

Proteins, Pulses & Nuts:

- Cashew nuts
- Chickpeas
- Eggs (white part only is acidic)
- Kidney beans
- Lentils
- Linseeds (flaxseeds)
- Macadamia nuts
- Peanuts
- Sesame seeds
- Sunflower seeds

Grains:

- Corn
- Buckwheat
- Millet
- Oats
- Quinoa
- Brown Rice
- Rye
- Spelt

Dairy:

- Feta cheese
- Goat's milk
- Halloumi cheese
- Fresh yogurt

Alkaline-Forming Foods List

The following is a list of beneficial alkaline-forming foods.

Fruits:

- Apples
- Apricots
- Avocados
- Blueberries
- Blackberries
- Cherries
- Dates
- Figs
- Grapefruit
- Grapes
- Guava
- Kiwi fruits
- Lemons
- Limes
- Mango
- Melons
- Olives
- Oranges
- Papaya
- Peaches
- Pears
- Pineapples
- Plums
- Raspberries
- Redcurrants
- Raisins
- Rhubarb
- Strawberries
- Sultanas
- Tomatoes (raw are more alkaline)

Vegetables:

- Alfalfa sprouts
- Artichokes
- Aubergines
- Asparagus
- Beetroot
- Broccoli
- Brussels Sprouts
- Cabbage
- Carrots
- Cauliflower

- Celery,
- Chicory
- Coconut
- Dandelion
- Endive lettuce
- Fennel
- Garlic
- Green beans
- Greens
- Horseradish
- Kale
- Kelp
- Kohlrabi
- Leek
- Lettuce
- Mange tout (Snow peas)
- Mushrooms
- Okra
- Onions
- Peas
- Peppers (bell peppers)
- Potatoes
- Pumpkin
- Radish
- Spinach
- Sprouted seeds
- Squash
- Sweetcorn
- Turnip
- Watercress
- Wheatgrass
- Goat's milk
- Halloumi cheese
- Fresh yogurt

Proteins:

- Black-eyed peas
- Butter beans
- Cannellini beans
- Haricot beans
- Soya beans
- Soya protein
- Tofu
- Nuts and seeds

Fats and Oils:

- Almond oil
- Coconut oil
- Groundnut oil
- Olive oil
- Sesame oil

Drinks:

- Almond milk
- Coconut water
- Coconut milk
- Herbal teas
- Soya milk

Condiments:

- Apple cider vinegar
- Cayenne pepper
- Chilli peppers
- Cumin
- Herbs
- Ginger
- Honey
- Lemongrass
- Mustard
- Sea salt or Himalayan salt
- Stevia
- Tamari
- Turmeric

7 Day Cleanse & Menu Plan

So when you begin your 7 day cleanse you should avoid all highly acid-forming foods. This may seem like you are being really strict with yourself, but bear in mind it is temporary and it gives your body a better chance to rest, balance and eliminate waste which has built up. So for one week, eat only alkaline or mildly-acidifying foods.

Avoid all meat, chicken, eggs, fish or shellfish, dairy produce (not even goat's milk produce during the first week). Avoid alcohol, caffeinated drinks, fizzy drinks (including carbonated water) and all sugar and products containing hidden sugars such as pre-prepared food, ketchup, sauces and chutneys.

Also, steer clear of very sweet fruit such as mangoes and figs to begin with due to the higher sugar content and opt for apples, grapefruits, avocados and lemons instead. In general, during the first week keep your fruit consumption low or avoid it completely to prevent you consuming too much fructose.

7 Day Cleanse Menu Plan

Day 1	Day 2	Day 3	Day 4	Day 5	Day 6	Day 7
Breakfast	**Breakfast**	**Breakfast**	**Breakfast**	**Breakfast**	**Breakfast**	**Breakfast**
Clean Green Smoothie	Carrot & Ginger Smoothie	Clean Green Smoothie	Fennel & Cucumber Smoothie	Clean Green Smoothie	Creamy Carrot Smoothie	Clean Green Smoothie
Lunch	**Lunch**	**Lunch**	**Lunch**	**Lunch**	**Lunch**	**Lunch**
Pumpkin & Potato Soup	Green Vegetable Soup	Stuffed Peppers	Kale & Butterbean Soup	Spicy Potato Cakes	Watercress Soup	Chestnut & Root Vegetable Stir-Fry
Dinner	**Dinner**	**Dinner**	**Dinner**	**Dinner**	**Dinner**	**Dinner**
Vegetable Bake	Fennel & Mushroom Casserole	Thai Green Curry Vegetables	Hot Pot	Vegetable Tagine	Cannellini Beans & Spinach	Mixed Vegetable Casserole
Drinks	**Drinks**	**Drinks**	**Drinks**	**Drinks**	**Drinks**	**Drinks**
Peppermint Tea Water	Chamomile Tea Water	Ginger Tea Water	Nettle Tea Water	Peppermint Tea Water	Nettle Tea Water	Ginger Tea Water

The 7 Day Cleanse menu plan is a guide to help you decide what to eat and you can interchange the foods depending on your preference. You might prefer to make a batch of soup and use that rather than make fresh soup daily. It's really whatever works best with your lifestyle. If you don't want to splash out on different ingredients every day you can repeat a smoothie or soup, just make sure you have greens daily.

The Everyday Alkaline Way

You have plenty of options for meal times and snacks. What you do need to bear in mind is the 80/20 rule. Your plate should consist of 80% alkaline foods and no more than 20% acid-forming. Once you get into the swing of it, you'll find you naturally stack your plate with ample vegetable based foods and that meat portions will have significantly reduced.

Can I Eat Meat?

Yes, you can but keep your meat consumption low and as with all acid-forming foods below 20% of your intake. If you're not a vegetarian, you can still eat meat. It's a good idea to have some meals which are totally plant based to make sure you stay well in the alkaline zone, plus you'll feel lighter and won't mentally be so dependent on the meat/protein component of your diet.

Chicken and fish are healthier options than red meat as they are easier to digest, so if you wish to combine alkaline foods with a small piece of poached salmon or grilled chicken you can. Eggs are a valuable source of protein and apart from being easy to combine into a healthy meal they can be hard-boiled and make a healthy snack to go alongside salads.

Following a highly alkaline diet is about reducing the acidic foods so that the majority of what you eat is alkaline-forming. If you can't always eat 80% alkaline just eat much as you can of that food group. If you're eating out try opting for salads or at least have vegetables and greens as an accompaniment. You don't need to cut out all food groups entirely and you want to ensure you get adequate nourishment. Just keep the balance to maintain the equilibrium in your body and aid your digestive system.

Top Tips

Making It Easier

- Stock up on alkaline foods that you know you like so you have staples in your cupboard.

- To avoid you getting the 'what can I eat' wobbles, prepare yourself some soup which can be kept refrigerated or stored in the freezer for such times.

- Stay hydrated! This is old news but it's still important. Drinking 4 pints of water a day is advisable. If you don't like it plain, flavour it with limes or lemons, or be adventurous and steep a small amount of other fruits, vegetables or herbs in a large jug to give it flavour.

- Digestion starts in your mouth so chew your food well. When we eat quickly it leaves more of the breakdown of our food to be done in the stomach, adding to its workload.

- Don't over-do it with lots of fruit. It does contain fructose which is a form of sugar. You could opt for lower sugar fruits instead. For instance grapes and figs have 16g of sugar per 100g which is high compared to raspberries which contain 4.4g per 100g and rhubarb which has only 1.1g.

- Have plenty of handy snacks available at work and carry them with you to fend off hunger and prevent you reaching for something quick and less healthy instead.

- Start your day with a large glass of water with a wedge of lemon squeezed into it. It's not only alkaline but it boosts your hydration first thing in the morning.

- Get some exercise every day. It doesn't need to be a hard-core gym workout, you can start off with 30 minutes walking every day. It'll boost your endorphins and take your mind off things if you get a longing for sugary food which could happen in the early part of your new healthy eating regime.

- Eating organic food is an added boost. It's not always possible to source it and it can be expensive. The important thing is to eat plenty of veggies.

- If you're finding eating the alkaline way challenging or you fall off the wagon, don't worry. Just do what you can without going crazy on the acidic foods. Keep going eating really good healthy alkaline foods. You don't have to be perfect. Easy does it.

- If you're doing the 7 day cleanse, avoid fruit and sweet recipes in this book, just to begin with. They can tempt your taste buds towards sweet foods and make it harder for you, plus fructose should be avoided in excess.

- Allow yourself occasional treats. No healthy diet should leave you feeling deprived. Knowing you have something tasty to look forward to can give you a boost and help you carry on.

- Always buffer acid-forming foods with alkaline-forming foods and you can adjust your eating depending on your health needs with a little of what you fancy.

- Reduce stress where possible and get plenty of sleep.

- Lastly, NO self-criticism. If negative self-judgement starts, nip it in the bud. This isn't about setting yourself impossibly high standards where you can berate or judge yourself for what you think you should have achieved. You've made a wonderful decision to improve your health and well-being which is to be applauded. Every step you take towards optimum health is a great achievement.

Frequently Asked Questions

Lemons and limes are acidic so how come I can eat these?

Lemons, like various other foods, are acidic but it's about the effect they have on the body. For instance dairy produce is alkaline and certainly hasn't an acidic taste however it has an acidic effect on the body. Foods which are alkaline before digestion can result in acidification and foods which are acidic before digestion can be alkalining inside the body.

Does doing the alkaline diet mean I should stop eating all acidifying foods?

No, it's all about balance. The key is to eat the right foods, which give you optimum nutrition and don't strain the body by eating foods which have little or no benefit to the body and make the body too acidic. Despite some foods being weakly acidifying, they still have nutritional benefits. Eggs are a great source of protein and fish is full of zinc and valuable omega oils. However, the nutritional content of junk food is negligible and/or harmful so it can be eradicated completely. If you are a meat eater or pesceterian you can still eat it keeping the 80/20 balance and eating plenty of greens to off-set the acids. The important thing is not to overwhelm the body with acidic foods which can hamper detoxification.

I've noticed conflicting information between alkaline diets about which foods are acid or alkaline. Why is this?

This is because even within food groups some foods are slightly more acidifying than others which makes classification difficult. That's why we've grouped the foods into 3 sections because some foods are weakly acidifying yet a nutritious form of nourishment and often a valuable source of plant based protein in the cases of pulses and nuts. So let's be sensible about this, adding pulses or healthy grains such as brown rice and quinoa are nowhere near as acidifying as a large steak, cakes, wine or coffee. Moderation is the key. For many eating just vegetables and fruits is too restrictive, nor does it provide you with a balanced diet.

What about alkaline water?

The pH levels of water vary and can fall into the acidic range. There are a great many products on the market which can be used to make water alkaline. Drops containing antioxidants and minerals can be added to water to help rid the body of toxicity and excess waste products by naturally supporting your body. They can greatly assist in rebalancing your body and neutralising the effects of acidic build up.

Add fresh lemon or lime juice to your drinking water to make it more alkaline. It's simple, cheap and easy.

Recipes

Eating The Alkaline Way

Once your taste buds have adjusted you'll be savouring a wide variety of subtler flavours with a range of vegetables in ample amounts. Some of the recipes in this book are for 1 person, especially the breakfast selection, because we know not everyone has the time to eat together and we often want something specific. Other meals are based on 4 people, so that these meals can either be shared or frozen and kept for another day. This can save you time later when you don't necessarily have a fridge full of ingredients or are hungry and stuck for something healthy to eat.

A good quality food processor or smoothie maker could be your best friend. If you haven't already got one you might want to think about investing in a good machine. There are numerous ones on the market at wide ranging prices. We find the Nutribullet to be reasonably priced, requires little cleaning and the smoothies are well blended and delicious.

So depending on what type of blender you have you can add nuts and seeds to your smoothies which will not only add protein to them but will keep you feeling fuller for longer and avoid hungry spells. If your blender doesn't allow for this you can buy ground flaxseeds or almonds and stir them into your drinks. Or you can add powdered spirulina or chlorella which is an algae used as a food supplement because it's high in protein and essential nutrients.

BREAKFAST

Fennel & Cucumber Smoothie

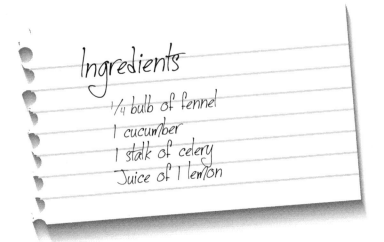

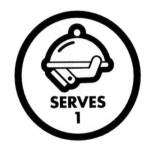

SERVES 1

Method

Place the fennel, cucumber and celery into a food processor or smoothie maker and add the lemon juice together with enough water to cover the ingredients. Process until smooth.

Clean Green Smoothie

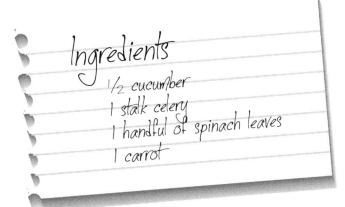

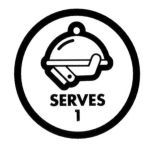

SERVES 1

Method

Put all the ingredients into a blender, and blitz until smooth. You can add ice to some blenders or crush some ice and add it to make your smoothie really refreshing.

Raspberry & Avocado Smoothie

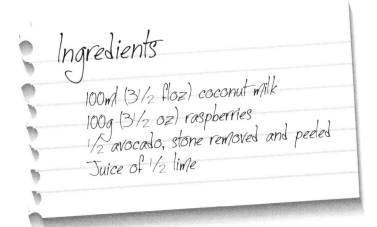

Ingredients

100ml (3½ floz) coconut milk
100g (3½ oz) raspberries
½ avocado, stone removed and peeled
Juice of ½ lime

SERVES
1

Method

Toss all of the ingredients into a blender. Blitz until creamy. If it seems too thick you can add some water. Pour and enjoy!

Carrot & Ginger Zinger

Ingredients

1-2 carrots
2 cm (1 inch) chunk fresh ginger
root, peeled
Juice of 1 lime

SERVES
1

Method

Place the carrots, ginger and lime juice into a blender with enough water to cover them. Blitz until smooth.

Summer Berry Smoothie

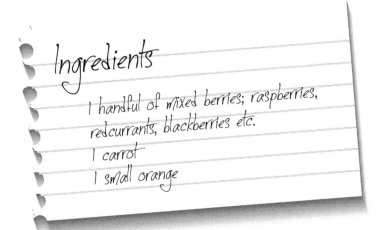

Ingredients

1 handful of mixed berries; raspberries, redcurrants, blackberries etc.
1 carrot
1 small orange

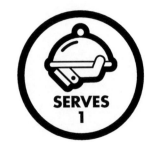

SERVES
1

Method

Place all the ingredients into a blender with enough water to cover them and process until smooth.

Kale & Apple Smoothie

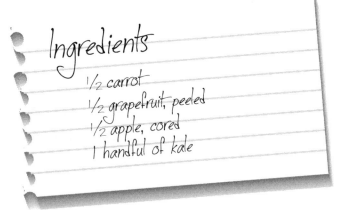

Ingredients

½ carrot
½ grapefruit, peeled
½ apple, cored
1 handful of kale

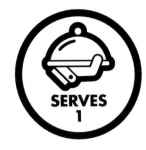

SERVES
1

Method

Place the ingredients into a blender with sufficient water to cover them and blitz until smooth.

Avocado & Carrot Smoothie

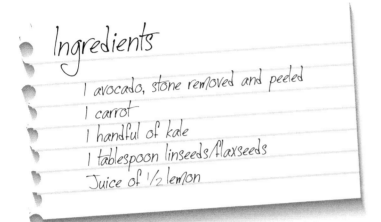

Ingredients

1 avocado, stone removed and peeled
1 carrot
1 handful of kale
1 tablespoon linseeds/flaxseeds
Juice of ½ lemon

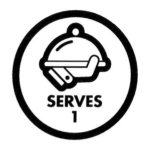

SERVES
1

Method

Place all the ingredients into a blender with enough water to cover and blitz until smooth.

Creamy Citrus Blend

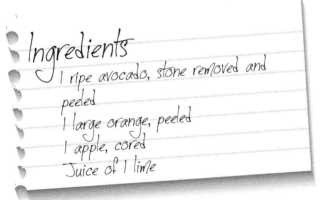

Ingredients

1 ripe avocado, stone removed and peeled
1 large orange, peeled
1 apple, cored
Juice of 1 lime

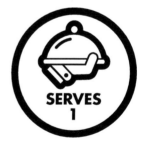

SERVES
1

Method

Place all the ingredients into a blender with enough water to cover and blitz until smooth.

Green Glory Smoothie

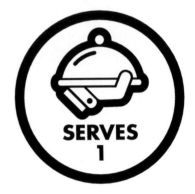

SERVES 1

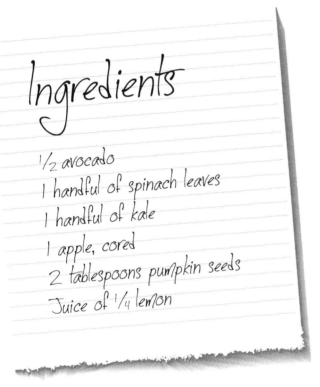

Ingredients

½ avocado
1 handful of spinach leaves
1 handful of kale
1 apple, cored
2 tablespoons pumpkin seeds
Juice of ¼ lemon

Method

Put all the ingredients into a blender with just enough water to cover them. Blitz until smooth. You can add more lemon juice for extra zing.

Blueberry Pancakes

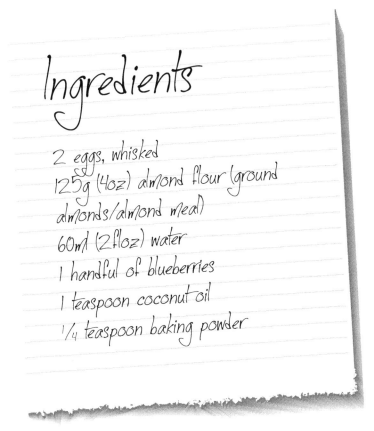

Ingredients

2 eggs, whisked
125g (4oz) almond flour (ground almonds/almond meal)
60ml (2 floz) water
1 handful of blueberries
1 teaspoon coconut oil
1/4 teaspoon baking powder

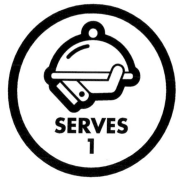

SERVES 1

Method

Combine the eggs, almond flour, water and baking powder in a bowl and mix until smooth. Heat the coconut oil in a frying pan. Pour some of the mixture into the pan and sprinkle some blueberries into the mixture while wet. Cook the pancakes until golden brown. You can top the pancakes with a little coconut oil and extra blueberries to garnish. Enjoy.

Quinoa & Berry Porridge

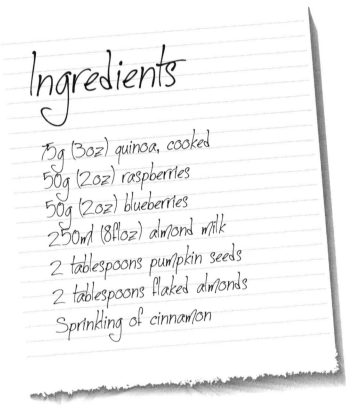

Ingredients

75g (3oz) quinoa, cooked
50g (2oz) raspberries
50g (2oz) blueberries
250ml (8floz) almond milk
2 tablespoons pumpkin seeds
2 tablespoons flaked almonds
Sprinkling of cinnamon

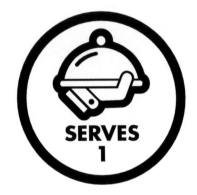

SERVES
1

Method

Place the quinoa and almond milk in a saucepan. Bring to the boil and cook for 5 minutes. Sprinkle in the cinnamon. Serve into a bowl, topped off with blueberries, pumpkin seeds and almonds.

Mixed Vegetable Omelette

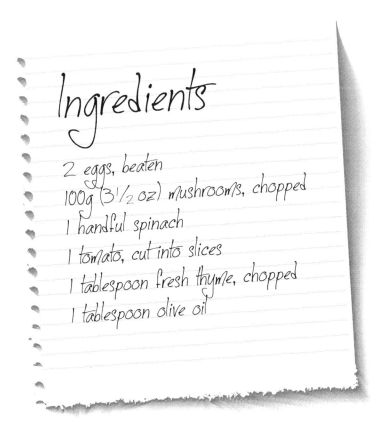

Ingredients

2 eggs, beaten
100g (3½ oz) mushrooms, chopped
1 handful spinach
1 tomato, cut into slices
1 tablespoon fresh thyme, chopped
1 tablespoon olive oil

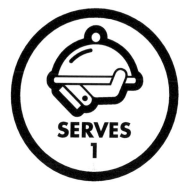

SERVES
1

Method

Heat the olive oil in a saucepan, add the mushrooms and cook until softened. Remove them and set aside. Pour the beaten eggs into the frying pan and allow them to set. Transfer the omelette to a plate and fill it with the mushrooms, spinach, tomato and herbs then fold it over. Enjoy.

Granola

Ingredients

- 150g (5oz) raw almonds, chopped
- 150g (5oz) raw walnuts, chopped
- 150g (5oz) raw pecans, chopped
- 75g (3oz) desiccated (shredded) coconut
- 75g (3oz) sunflower seeds
- 75g (3oz) sultanas or raisins
- 75g (3oz) ground linseed/flaxseed or flaxseed meal
- 120ml (4floz) coconut oil
- 2 tablespoons honey
- 1/2 teaspoon sea salt

Method

Grease and line a baking sheet with grease-proof paper. Melt the coconut oil and mix it with the honey. Add it to the nuts, coconut, seeds and salt. Mix it together in a bowl and turn out onto the baking sheet. Scatter the granola evenly. Bake at 150C/300F for 30-40 minutes. During baking stir the mixture once or twice to make sure it bakes evenly. Cook until slightly golden. Allow it to cool then add in the sultanas and store in an airtight container. Serve the granola with almond milk or nibble on it as a snack.

Leek & Potato Frittata

Ingredients

250g (9oz) new potatoes

6 eggs

200g (7oz) fresh or frozen peas

1 large or 2 small leeks, roughly chopped

2 tablespoons fresh chives, chopped

2 tablespoons fresh parsley, chopped

120ml (4 floz) almond milk

2 tablespoons olive oil

Sea salt

Freshly ground pepper

SERVES 4

Method

Boil the potatoes until tender then drain them. Heat the oil in a frying pan and add the leeks and peas. Cook until the leeks have softened and the peas are warmed through. Dice the potatoes and add them to the frying pan. In a bowl whisk together the eggs and almond milk then sprinkle in the herbs and stir well. Season with salt and pepper. Pour the egg mixture into the frying pan containing the vegetables and make sure the mixture completely covers the pan. Allow the eggs to firm up. Place the frying pan under a preheated grill (broiler) and cook for 2-3 minutes until the top of the frittata is golden. Serve and enjoy.

LUNCH

Pumpkin & Potato Soup

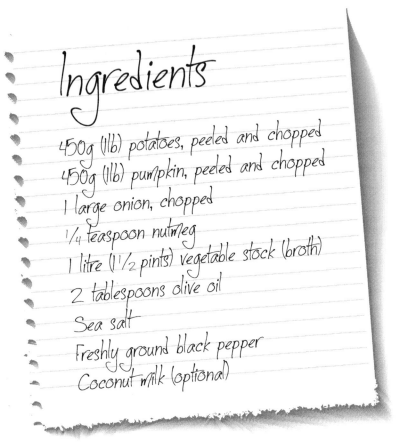

Ingredients

450g (1lb) potatoes, peeled and chopped
450g (1lb) pumpkin, peeled and chopped
1 large onion, chopped
1/4 teaspoon nutmeg
1 litre (1½ pints) vegetable stock (broth)
2 tablespoons olive oil
Sea salt
Freshly ground black pepper
Coconut milk (optional)

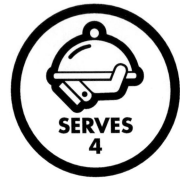

SERVES 4

Method

Heat the olive oil in a saucepan, add the onion and cook until slightly softened. Stir in the pumpkin and potatoes and cook for 5 minutes. Pour in the stock (broth) and sprinkle in the nutmeg. Bring to the boil, reduce the heat and simmer for 20 minutes until the vegetables are tender. Using a hand blender or food processor blend the soup until smooth. Season with salt and pepper then serve. If you like your soup extra creamy, try adding some coconut milk towards the end of cooking.

Cream Of Mushroom Soup

Ingredients

SERVES 4-6

450g (1lb) mushrooms, chopped
1 large leek, finely chopped
1 tablespoon cornflour (cornstarch)
750ml (1¼ pints) vegetable stock (broth)
400ml (14fl oz) almond milk
3 tablespoons olive oil
Juice of 1 lemon
Sea salt
Freshly ground black pepper

Method

Heat the olive oil in a saucepan. Add the leek and mushrooms and cook for 8 minutes or until the vegetables are soft. Sprinkle in the cornflour (cornstarch) and stir. Pour in the almond milk together with the stock (broth). Bring to the boil, cover and simmer gently for 30 minutes. Using a hand blender or food processor, blend the soup until smooth. Return to the heat if necessary. Stir in the lemon juice and season with salt and pepper just before serving.

Potato & Leek Soup

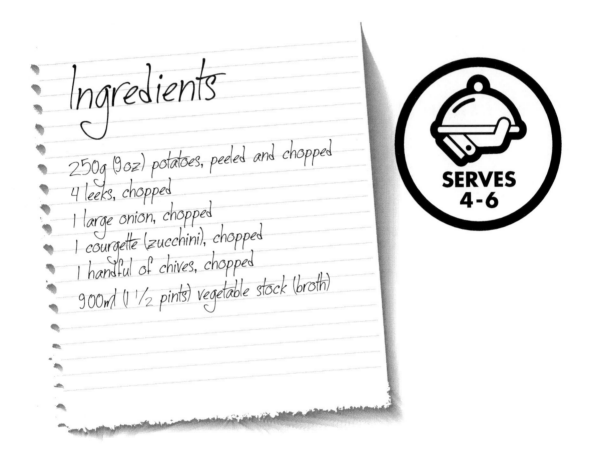

Ingredients

250g (9oz) potatoes, peeled and chopped
4 leeks, chopped
1 large onion, chopped
1 courgette (zucchini), chopped
1 handful of chives, chopped
900ml (1 ½ pints) vegetable stock (broth)

SERVES 4-6

Method

Heat the stock (broth) in a saucepan and add the vegetables but not including the chives. Reduce the heat and simmer for 15 minutes. Remove the soup from the heat and blend using a food processor or hand blender until smooth. Serve into bowls and sprinkle with chives.

Miso Broth

SERVES 4

Ingredients

225g (8oz) pak choi (bok choy), chopped
200g (7oz) tofu, cubed
10 spring onions (scallions), finely chopped
2 star anise
3 tablespoons red miso
1 tablespoon fresh coriander (cilantro), chopped
1 cm (½ inch) piece of fresh ginger root, very finely chopped
1 small red chilli pepper
1200ml (2 pints) vegetable stock (broth)
2 tablespoons tamari sauce

Method

Place the pak choi (bok choy) into a saucepan with the ginger, star anise, coriander, chilli and vegetable stock (broth). Bring to the boil, reduce the heat and simmer for 10 minutes. Add the spring onions (scallions), tamari sauce and tofu. Cook for 3-4 minutes. In a bowl, mix together the red miso with a few tablespoons of the soup then stir the miso into the soup. Add in the coriander (cilantro) and cook for 1 minute, making sure the soup is warm through. Serve into bowls.

Celeriac & Apple Soup

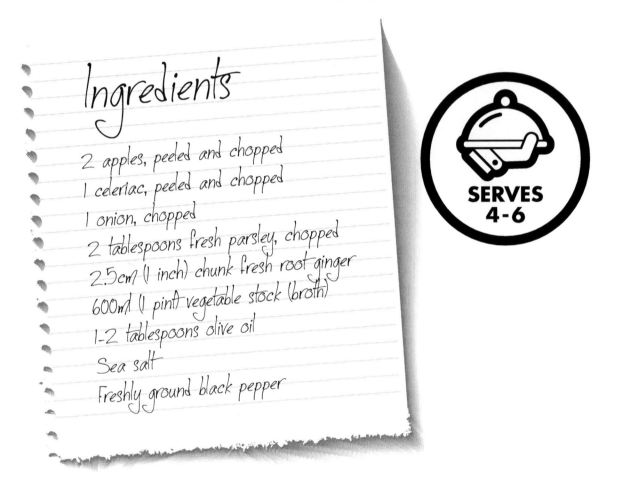

Ingredients

2 apples, peeled and chopped
1 celeriac, peeled and chopped
1 onion, chopped
2 tablespoons fresh parsley, chopped
2.5cm (1 inch) chunk fresh root ginger
600ml (1 pint) vegetable stock (broth)
1-2 tablespoons olive oil
Sea salt
Freshly ground black pepper

SERVES 4-6

Method

Heat the olive oil in a saucepan, add the onion, celeriac, apples, ginger and cook for 5 minutes. Pour in the stock (broth) bring to the boil, reduce the heat and cook for 20-25 minutes. Use a hand blender or food processor and blitz until smooth. You can add extra stock or hot water to make it thinner if you wish. Sprinkle in the parsley and season with salt and pepper.

Green Vegetable Soup

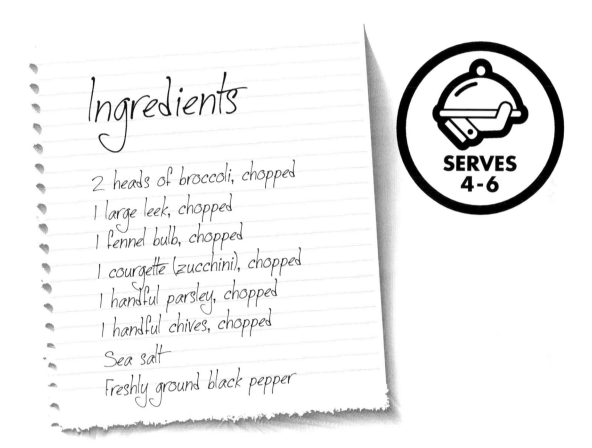

Ingredients

2 heads of broccoli, chopped

1 large leek, chopped

1 fennel bulb, chopped

1 courgette (zucchini), chopped

1 handful parsley, chopped

1 handful chives, chopped

Sea salt

Freshly ground black pepper

SERVES 4-6

Method

Place the broccoli, leek, courgette (zucchini) and fennel in enough water to cover them and bring to the boil. Simmer for 10-15 minutes or until the vegetables are tender. Stir in the herbs. Using a hand blender or food processor blend until the soup becomes smooth. Add more water if required to adjust the consistency. Season and serve.

Roasted Red Pepper Soup (Bell pepper)

Ingredients

4 red peppers (Bell peppers)
1 small onion, chopped
2 cloves of garlic crushed
1 large tomato, chopped
1 carrot, chopped
600ml (1 pint) vegetable stock (broth)
600ml (1 pint) water
1 tablespoon olive oil
Sea salt
Freshly ground black pepper

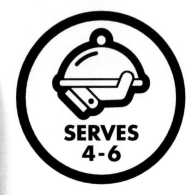

SERVES 4-6

Method

Heat a grill (broiler) and place the peppers (Bell peppers) underneath. Keep turning them until the skin becomes charred on all sides. Remove them from the heat and carefully remove the skins, seeds and stalks then set aside. Heat the oil in a saucepan and add the onion and garlic. Cook for 4 minutes. Add in the tomatoes, carrot, red peppers, water and stock (broth). Bring to the boil, reduce the heat and simmer for 20 minutes. Use a hand blender or food processor and blitz the soup until smooth. Season with salt and pepper. Serve and enjoy.

Watercress Soup

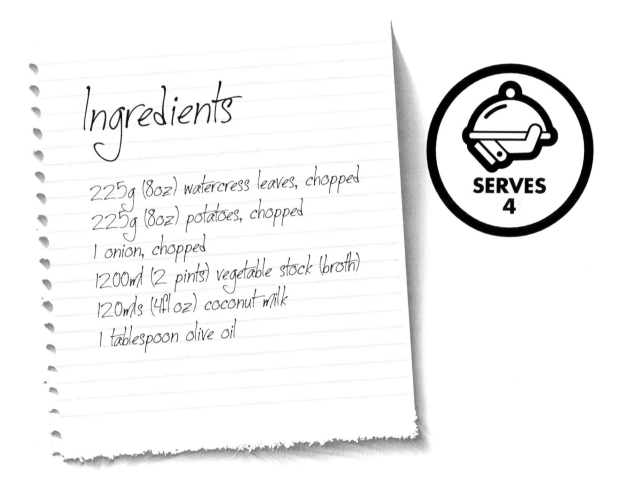

Ingredients

225g (8oz) watercress leaves, chopped
225g (8oz) potatoes, chopped
1 onion, chopped
1200ml (2 pints) vegetable stock (broth)
120mls (4fl oz) coconut milk
1 tablespoon olive oil

SERVES 4

Method

Heat the olive oil in a saucepan, add the onion and cook 4 minutes. Add the potatoes and stock (broth). Bring to the boil, reduce the heat and simmer for 15 minutes. Add the watercress and cook for 5 minutes. Remove from the heat. Using a hand blender or food processor, process the soup until smooth. Pour in the coconut milk, re-heat the soup and serve.

Kale & Butterbean Soup

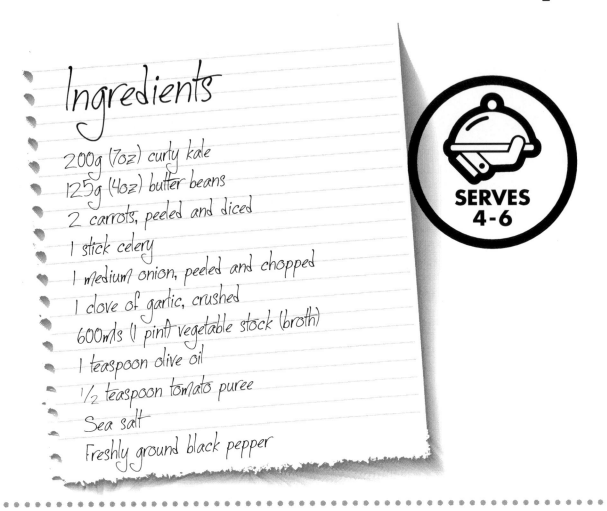

Ingredients

- 200g (7oz) curly kale
- 125g (4oz) butter beans
- 2 carrots, peeled and diced
- 1 stick celery
- 1 medium onion, peeled and chopped
- 1 clove of garlic, crushed
- 600mls (1 pint) vegetable stock (broth)
- 1 teaspoon olive oil
- ½ teaspoon tomato puree
- Sea salt
- Freshly ground black pepper

SERVES 4-6

Method

Heat the olive oil in a large saucepan and add all of the vegetables apart from the kale and butterbeans. Stir for 2-3 minutes on a medium heat. Add the stock (broth) and bring to boil. Reduce and cook for 15 minutes. Blend half the butter beans and add to the soup. Add the kale, the remaining butter beans, tomato puree and cook for 10 minutes. This soup can be blended smooth or left chunky if you prefer. Season with salt and pepper then serve.

Beetroot Soup

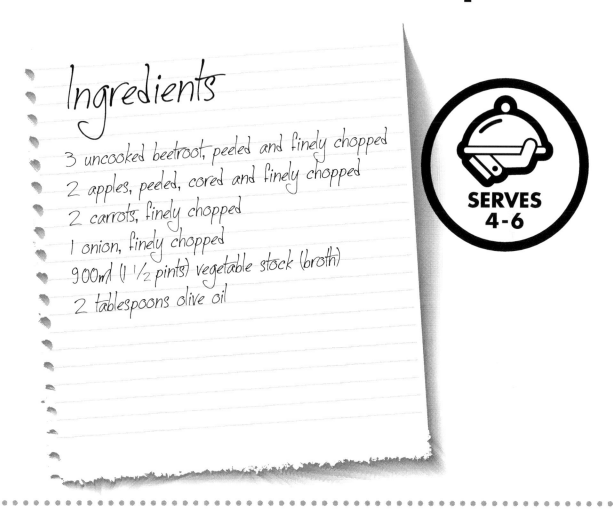

Ingredients

3 uncooked beetroot, peeled and finely chopped

2 apples, peeled, cored and finely chopped

2 carrots, finely chopped

1 onion, finely chopped

900ml (1½ pints) vegetable stock (broth)

2 tablespoons olive oil

SERVES 4-6

Method

Place the oil in a saucepan and add the onion. Cook for 4 minutes until it softens. Add in the beetroot and carrots to the saucepan and cook for 15 minutes. Add in the stock (broth) and apples. Bring to the boil, reduce the heat and simmer for 20 minutes. Blend the soup until smooth or serve as it is. Pour into bowls and enjoy.

Winter Vegetable & Lentil Soup

Ingredients

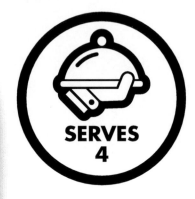

SERVES 4

75g (3oz) lentils
2 sticks of celery, chopped
2 cloves of garlic, chopped
2 potatoes, chopped
2 carrots, chopped
2 tablespoons fresh parsley, chopped
1 parsnip, chopped
1 red onion, chopped
1 sweet potato, chopped
1 bay leaf
900ml (1 ½ pints) vegetable stock (broth)
Extra parsley to garnish

Method

Place the stock (broth) into a saucepan, bring to the boil and reduce the heat. Stir in the vegetables, lentils and the bay leaf. Simmer for 30 minutes until the vegetables are tender. Remove the bay leaf. Using a hand blender, process until it's only partially blended, leaving it thick and chunky. Sprinkle with parsley and serve.

Fennel, Lime & Butterbean Soup

Ingredients

400g (14oz) butter beans
2 large fennel bulbs
1 carrot, chopped
1 onion, chopped
1 courgette, chopped
1 clove of garlic, chopped
900ml (1 ½ pints) vegetable stock (broth)
Sea salt
Freshly ground black pepper

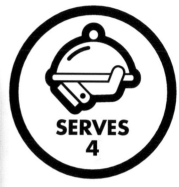

SERVES 4

Method

Heat the vegetable stock (broth) in a large saucepan. Add in all of the vegetables but not the butterbeans just yet. Bring them to the boil, reduce the heat and simmer for 20 minutes. Add the butterbeans and stir until warmed through. Using a hand blender or food processor, process the soup until smooth. Season and serve.

Spiced Butternut Squash Soup

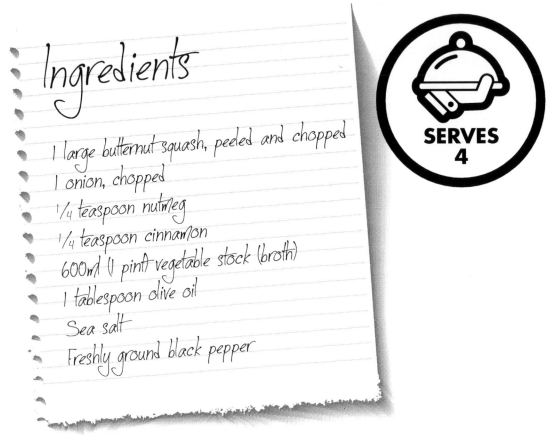

Ingredients

1 large butternut squash, peeled and chopped
1 onion, chopped
1/4 teaspoon nutmeg
1/4 teaspoon cinnamon
600ml (1 pint) vegetable stock (broth)
1 tablespoon olive oil
Sea salt
Freshly ground black pepper

SERVES 4

Method

Bring the stock in a large saucepan and add the squash and onion. Bring to the boil, reduce the heat and simmer for 30 minutes. Sprinkle in the cinnamon and nutmeg. Transfer to a food processor or use a hand blender and blitz until smooth. Season with salt and pepper. If you prefer to add some extra nutmeg and cinnamon you can sprinkle it in and stir. Serve and enjoy..

Crudités & Aubergine Dip

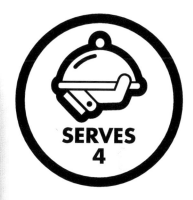

SERVES 4

Ingredients

For the dip:
1 aubergine (eggplant), chopped
3 tablespoons toasted sesame seeds
1 red chilli
1 teaspoons sesame oil
Juice of ½ lime
Sea salt
Freshly ground black pepper

For the crudités:
125g (4oz) broccoli florets
125g (4oz) cauliflower florets
2 carrots, cut into batons
3 sticks of celery, cut into batons
1 romaine lettuce, cut into slices

Method

Steam the aubergine (eggplant) for around 6 minutes, or until soft. Allow to cool. Place the sesame seeds, cooked aubergine, chilli, sesame oil and lime juice into a food processor or blender and process until the mixture is fairly smooth. Season with salt and pepper to taste. Spoon the dip into a bowl. Serve the crudités on a plate, dip and enjoy.

Fennel Salad

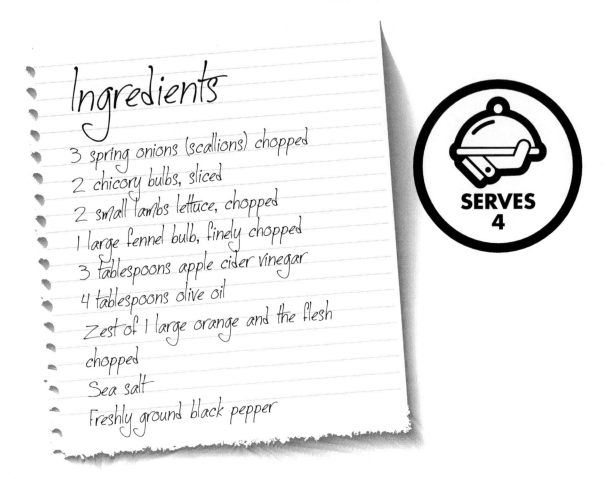

Ingredients

3 spring onions (scallions) chopped

2 chicory bulbs, sliced

2 small lambs lettuce, chopped

1 large fennel bulb, finely chopped

3 tablespoons apple cider vinegar

4 tablespoons olive oil

Zest of 1 large orange and the flesh chopped

Sea salt

Freshly ground black pepper

SERVES 4

Method

Place the lettuce, chicory and spring onion (scallion) into a bowl. In a separate bowl mix together the olive oil, vinegar and orange zest. Mix the dressing well and season with salt and pepper. Place the fennel and orange flesh into the dressing and mix well. Pour the dressing, fennel and orange over the salad and toss it. Chill before serving.

Lemon Lentil Salad

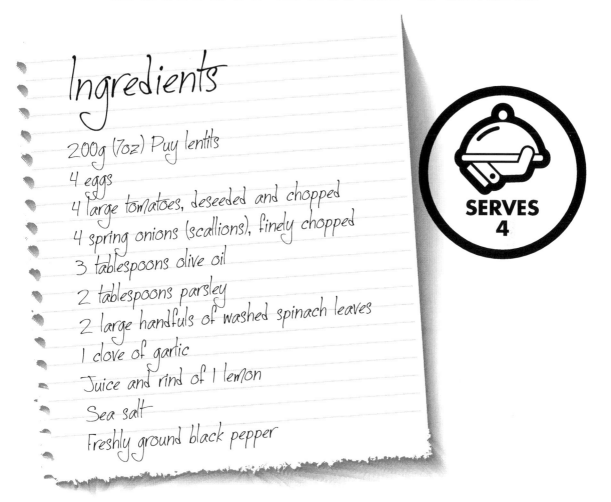

Ingredients

200g (7oz) Puy lentils

4 eggs

4 large tomatoes, deseeded and chopped

4 spring onions (scallions), finely chopped

3 tablespoons olive oil

2 tablespoons parsley

2 large handfuls of washed spinach leaves

1 clove of garlic

Juice and rind of 1 lemon

Sea salt

Freshly ground black pepper

SERVES 4

Method

Place the lentils in a saucepan, cover them with water and bring them to the boil. Reduce the heat and cook for 20-25 minutes. Drain them once they are soft. Heat the olive oil in a saucepan, add the garlic and spring onions (scallions) and cook for 2 minutes. Stir in the tomatoes, lemon juice and rind. Cook for 2 minutes. Stir in the lentils and keep warm. In a pan of gently simmering water, poach the eggs until they are set but soft in the middle which should be 3-4 minutes. Scatter the spinach leaves onto plates, serve the lentils and top off with a poached egg. Season with salt and pepper.

Celeriac & Carrot Mash

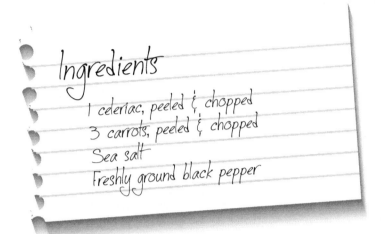

Ingredients

1 celeriac, peeled & chopped
3 carrots, peeled & chopped
Sea salt
Freshly ground black pepper

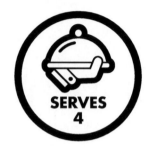

SERVES
4

Method

Place the vegetables in a saucepan of cold water. Bring to the boil and simmer for 20 minutes. Drain the celeriac and carrots then mash them. Season with salt and pepper.

Lemon Baked Asparagus

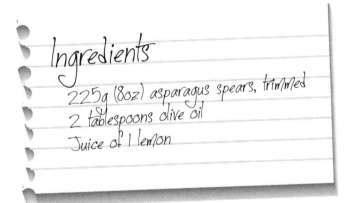

Ingredients

225g (8oz) asparagus spears, trimmed
2 tablespoons olive oil
Juice of 1 lemon

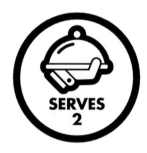

SERVES
2

Method

Lay out the asparagus spears on a baking tray. Mix together the olive oil and lemon juice then pour it over the asparagus. Place it in the oven at 200C/400F for 12 minutes, turning the asparagus over half way through cooking. Serve and eat.

Avocado & Melon Salad

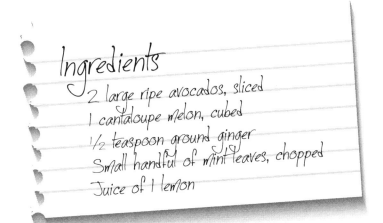

Ingredients
2 large ripe avocados, sliced
1 cantaloupe melon, cubed
½ teaspoon ground ginger
Small handful of mint leaves, chopped
Juice of 1 lemon

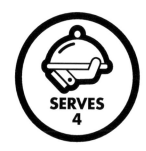

SERVES 4

Method

Mix the lemon juice, ginger and mint leaves together in a bowl. Add the avocados and melon and toss gently. Chill before serving.

Roast Pepper & Feta Salad

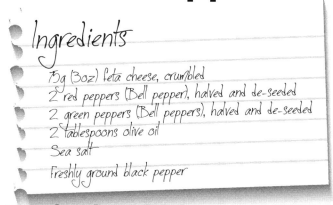

Ingredients
75g (3oz) feta cheese, crumbled
2 red peppers (Bell pepper), halved and de-seeded
2 green peppers (Bell peppers), halved and de-seeded
2 tablespoons olive oil
Sea salt
Freshly ground black pepper

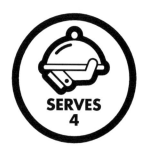

SERVES 4

Method

Place the peppers under a hot grill (broiler) until the skins begins to blacken. Remove them and place them inside a plastic bag for several minutes to help loosen the skin. Peel off skin and transfer the peppers to a serving plate. Drizzle with olive oil and sprinkle with feta cheese. Season with salt and pepper.

Quinoa Salad

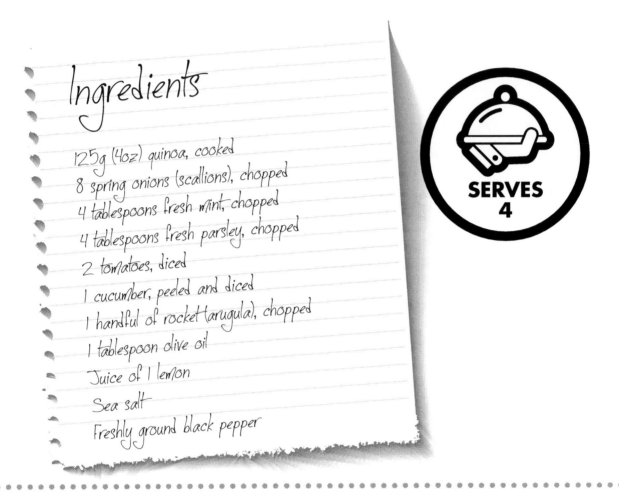

Ingredients

125g (4oz) quinoa, cooked
8 spring onions (scallions), chopped
4 tablespoons fresh mint, chopped
4 tablespoons fresh parsley, chopped
2 tomatoes, diced
1 cucumber, peeled and diced
1 handful of rocket (arugula), chopped
1 tablespoon olive oil
Juice of 1 lemon
Sea salt
Freshly ground black pepper

SERVES 4

Method

Combine all of the ingredients in a large bowl and mix well. Season with salt and pepper. Cover and place in the fridge for 20 minutes to chill before serving.

Warm Macadamia Salad

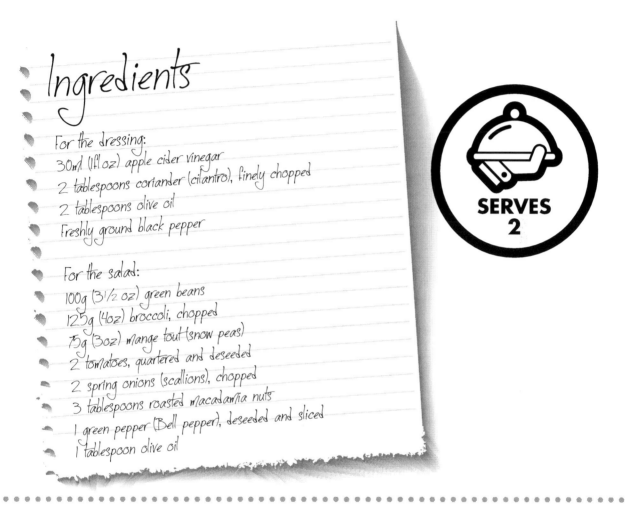

Ingredients

For the dressing:
30ml (1fl oz) apple cider vinegar
2 tablespoons coriander (cilantro), finely chopped
2 tablespoons olive oil
Freshly ground black pepper

For the salad:
100g (3½ oz) green beans
125g (4oz) broccoli, chopped
75g (3oz) mange tout (snow peas)
2 tomatoes, quartered and deseeded
2 spring onions (scallions), chopped
3 tablespoons roasted macadamia nuts
1 green pepper (Bell pepper), deseeded and sliced
1 tablespoon olive oil

SERVES 2

Method

For the dressing, combine the olive oil, vinegar and thyme in a bowl and mix well. Season with black pepper. For the salad, heat a tablespoon of olive oil in a frying pan. Add the green beans, broccoli, mange tout (snow peas) and green pepper (bell pepper). Stir and cook for 3 minutes. Add the tomatoes and spring onions (scallions) and heat through. Coat the vegetables in the dressing. Serve into bowls and sprinkle with macadamia nuts.

Herby Broad Bean Salad

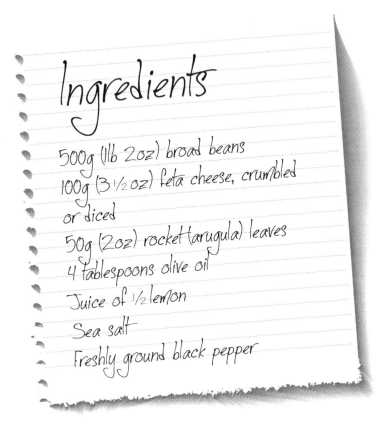

Ingredients

500g (1lb 2oz) broad beans
100g (3½oz) feta cheese, crumbled or diced
50g (2oz) rocket (arugula) leaves
4 tablespoons olive oil
Juice of ½ lemon
Sea salt
Freshly ground black pepper

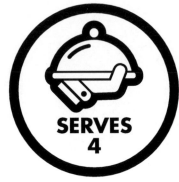

SERVES 4

Method

Cook the beans in boiling water for around 3 minutes until they are tender. Drain them, dip them in cool water then set aside and make sure they are properly drained. Combine the feta cheese in a bowl with the rocket (arugula) leaves and cold broad beans. Pour on the olive oil and squeeze on the lemon juice. Season with salt and pepper. Chill and serve.

Greek Salad

Ingredients

450g (1lb) tomatoes, chopped into eighths
125g (4oz) feta cheese, crumbled
50g (2oz) pitted black olives, halved
1 romaine lettuce, finely chopped
1 cucumber, deseeded and chopped

Dressing:
3 tablespoons olive oil
Juice of ½ lemon
Sea salt
Freshly ground black pepper

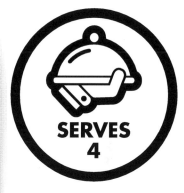

SERVES 4

Method

Place all the salad ingredients into a bowl. In a separate bowl, mix together the ingredients for the dressing. Pour the dressing into the salad and toss it well before serving.

Stuffed Peppers

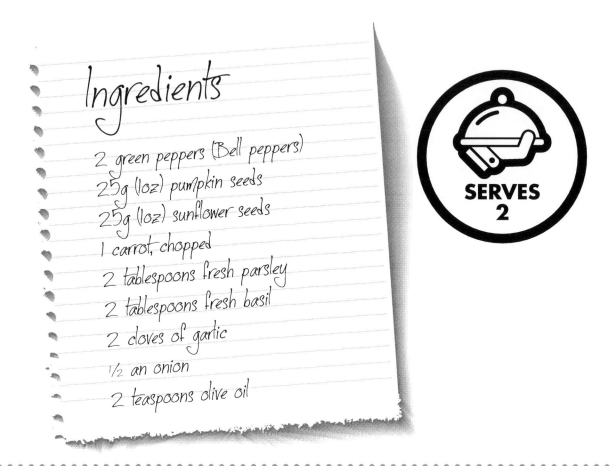

Ingredients

2 green peppers (Bell peppers)
25g (1oz) pumpkin seeds
25g (1oz) sunflower seeds
1 carrot, chopped
2 tablespoons fresh parsley
2 tablespoons fresh basil
2 cloves of garlic
1/2 an onion
2 teaspoons olive oil

SERVES 2

Method

Put the carrot, seeds, garlic, herbs, olive oil and onion into a blender and blitz until it is well combined. Cut the peppers in half and remove and discard the seeds. Stuff the peppers with the seed mixture. Place on a baking sheet, transfer to the oven and bake at 180C/350F for 20 minutes.

Polenta Pizza

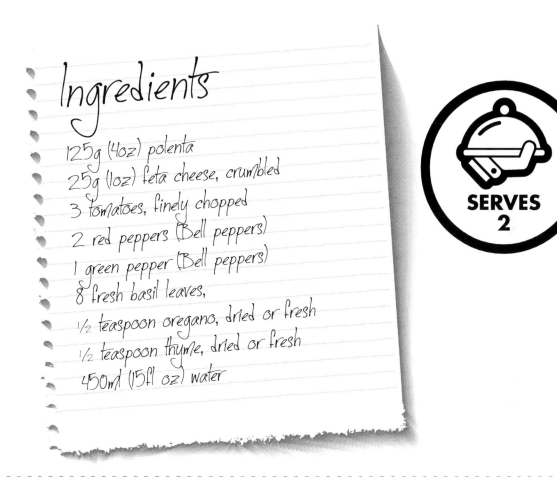

Ingredients

125g (4oz) polenta
25g (1oz) feta cheese, crumbled
3 tomatoes, finely chopped
2 red peppers (Bell peppers)
1 green pepper (Bell peppers)
8 fresh basil leaves,
1/2 teaspoon oregano, dried or fresh
1/2 teaspoon thyme, dried or fresh
450ml (15fl oz) water

SERVES 2

Method

Cut the peppers (bell peppers) in half and remove the seeds. Place the peppers under a grill (broiler) with the skin facing upwards. Cook them until they begin to blacken. Remove them and place them inside a plastic bag for a few minutes until the skin loosens, then peel it off. Bring the water to the boil and pour in the polenta together with the thyme and oregano. Stir and cook for around 8 minutes or until the polenta becomes thick. Grease a baking sheet and pour the polenta onto it. Spread it into a circular pizza shape. Chop the roasted peppers and place them on the polenta base together with the chopped tomatoes and basil leaves. Sprinkle over the feta cheese. Bake in the oven for around 14 minutes. Serve and eat straight away.

Spicy Sweet Potato Cakes

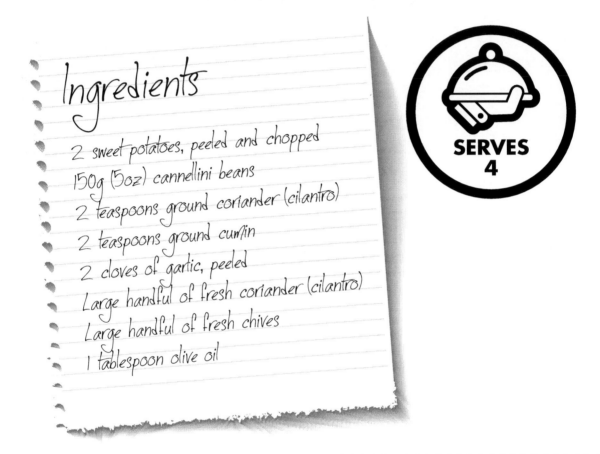

SERVES 4

Ingredients

2 sweet potatoes, peeled and chopped

150g (5oz) cannellini beans

2 teaspoons ground coriander (cilantro)

2 teaspoons ground cumin

2 cloves of garlic, peeled

Large handful of fresh coriander (cilantro)

Large handful of fresh chives

1 tablespoon olive oil

Method

Steam the sweet potato until soft and tender. Set it aside until it cools down. Place all of the ingredients, apart from the olive oil, into a food processor and blitz until you have everything is combined. Shape the mixture into patties then place them in the fridge for an hour to become firm. Grease a baking tray with the olive oil. Place the sweet potato cakes onto the tray and bake in the oven at 220C/440F for around 15 minutes or until slightly golden.

Chestnut & Root Vegetable Stir-Fry

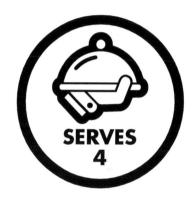

SERVES 4

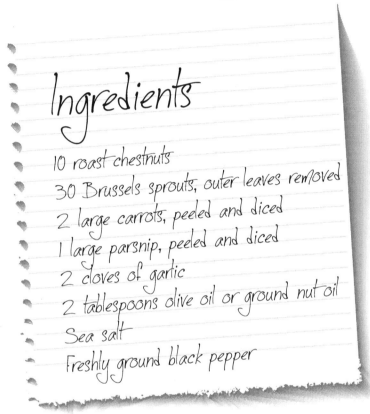

Ingredients

10 roast chestnuts

30 Brussels sprouts, outer leaves removed

2 large carrots, peeled and diced

1 large parsnip, peeled and diced

2 cloves of garlic

2 tablespoons olive oil or ground nut oil

Sea salt

Freshly ground black pepper

Method

Steam the Brussels sprouts for around 5 minutes then dip them in cold water to prevent them over-cooking. Set aside. Place the oil in a wok or frying pan and add parsnip, carrots and garlic. Cook for around 5 minutes until the parsnip and carrots are tender. Add the Brussels sprouts and chestnuts to the pan and heat them thoroughly. Season with salt and pepper before serving.

Beetroot & Orange Salad

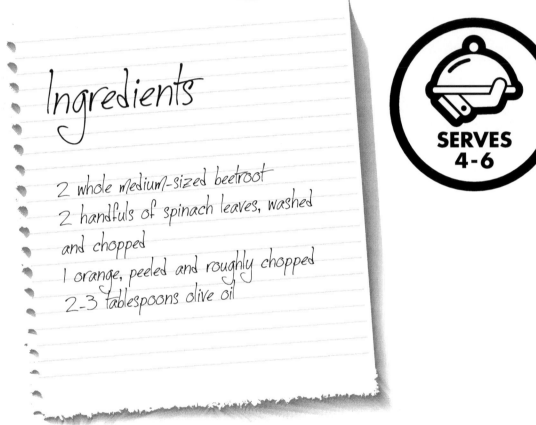

SERVES 4-6

Ingredients

2 whole medium-sized beetroot
2 handfuls of spinach leaves, washed
and chopped
1 orange, peeled and roughly chopped
2-3 tablespoons olive oil

Method

Place the whole beetroot on a baking tray and coat with a tablespoon of olive oil. Bake in the oven at 200C/400F for 45 minutes. Allow to cool. Peel and dice the beetroot. Place it in a bowl with the orange pieces and spinach leaves. Drizzle over 1-2 tablespoons olive oil and toss the salad before serving.

Walnut & Almond Salad

Ingredients

225g (8oz) bean sprouts
100g (3 ½ oz) almonds, finely chopped
1 cucumber, grated (shredded)
1-2 large carrots, grated (shredded)
Handful of fresh coriander (cilantro)

For the dressing:
1 clove of garlic, crushed
2 tablespoons tamari sauce
2 tablespoons honey
Juice of 1 lemon

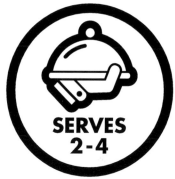

**SERVES
2-4**

Method

Combine the cucumber, carrots, bean sprouts and almonds in a bowl. In a separate container, mix together the garlic, tamari sauce, honey and lemon juice. Pour the dressing onto the salad vegetables, sprinkle with coriander (cilantro) and serve.

Avocado & Black-Eyed Pea Salad

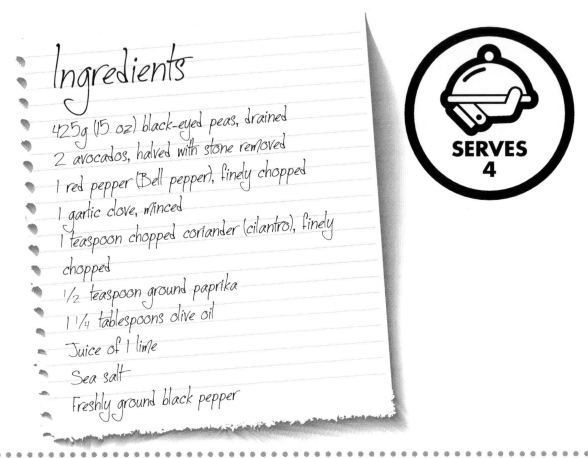

Ingredients

425g (15 oz) black-eyed peas, drained
2 avocados, halved with stone removed
1 red pepper (Bell pepper), finely chopped
1 garlic clove, minced
1 teaspoon chopped coriander (cilantro), finely chopped
1/2 teaspoon ground paprika
1 1/4 tablespoons olive oil
Juice of 1 lime
Sea salt
Freshly ground black pepper

SERVES 4

Method

To make the dressing, put the lime juice in a large bowl and whisk in the olive oil. Stir in the black-eyed peas, red pepper (Bell pepper), coriander (cilantro), garlic, paprika, salt and black pepper. Mix together until everything is coated with the dressing. Place the avocado halves on 4 plates. Spoon the mixture over the avocado and serve.

Roast Garlic & Spinach Salad

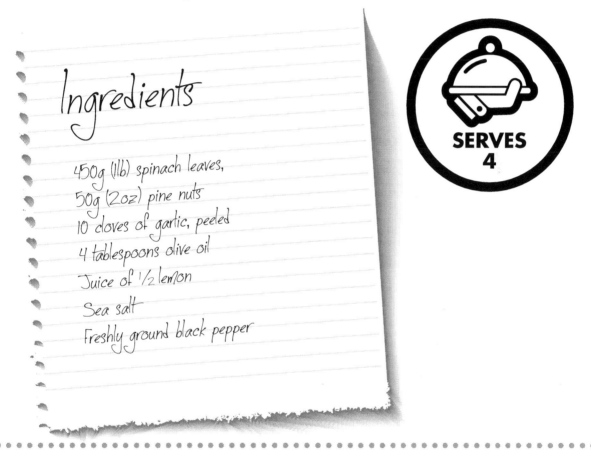

SERVES 4

Ingredients

450g (1lb) spinach leaves,
50g (2oz) pine nuts
10 cloves of garlic, peeled
4 tablespoons olive oil
Juice of ½ lemon
Sea salt
Freshly ground black pepper

Method

Place the garlic cloves on a baking tray and completely coat them in 2 tablespoons of olive oil. Bake in the oven at 190C/375F for 10 minutes. Place the spinach, lemon juice, pine nuts and olive oil into a bowl and combine. Add in the roast garlic and season with salt and pepper. Serve and eat immediately.

Black Bean & Pumpkin Salad

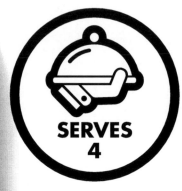

SERVES 4

Ingredients

400g (14oz) pumpkin, peeled and cubed
400g (14oz) black beans, drained
4 spring onions (scallions) chopped
2 tablespoons fresh chives, chopped
1 large onion, finely chopped
1 tablespoon fresh parsley, chopped
1 tablespoon olive oil

Dressing
2 tablespoons olive oil
1 teaspoon paprika
Small handful of basil leaves
Juice of 1 lemon

Method

Steam the pumpkin until tender and set aside. Heat the oil in a saucepan. Add the onion and pumpkin and cook for 5 minutes. Transfer it to a large serving bowl. Add the black beans, spring onions and herbs and combine. Mix together all of the ingredients for the dressing and stir it into the salad before serving.

DINNER

Vegetable Bake

Ingredients

650g (1 ½ lb) potatoes, thinly and evenly sliced
2 large leeks, thinly sliced
2 red peppers (Bell peppers), sliced
2 cloves of garlic, crushed
1 courgette (zucchini), sliced
1 handful of parsley, chopped
300mls (½ pint) vegetable stock (broth)
Olive oil for greasing

SERVES 4

Method

Grease a large casserole dish with olive oil. Place a layer of potatoes on the bottom of the casserole dish and sprinkle a little parsley on top. Add a layer of leeks, followed by a layer of courgette (zucchini), peppers (Bell peppers), garlic and parsley. Place a layer of potatoes on top and repeat until all the vegetables have been used up. Pour on the vegetable stock (broth). Bake in the oven at 180C/360F for 90 minutes until the top is golden.

Potato & Broccoli Hash

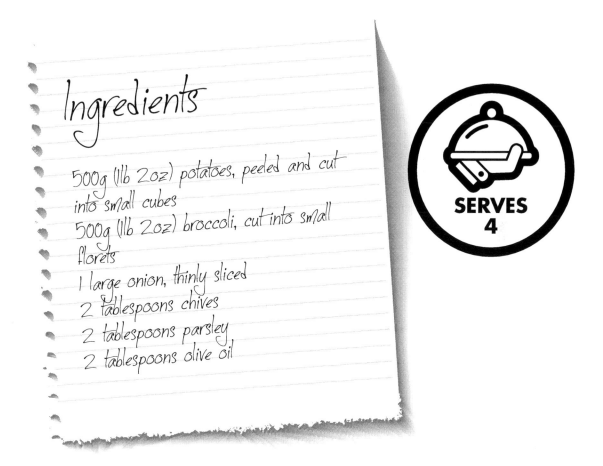

Ingredients

500g (1lb 2oz) potatoes, peeled and cut into small cubes
500g (1lb 2oz) broccoli, cut into small florets
1 large onion, thinly sliced
2 tablespoons chives
2 tablespoons parsley
2 tablespoons olive oil

SERVES 4

Method

Boil the potatoes until soft and tender. In the meantime add the broccoli to a steamer and cook for another 4 minutes. Heat the oil in a frying pan. Add the onion and cook until soft. Add the broccoli and potatoes to the pan and stir until crisp. Sprinkle in the herbs before serving.

Cabbage & Leek Stir-Fry

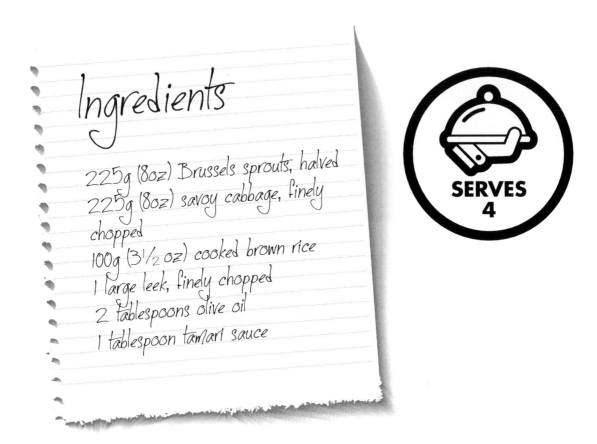

Ingredients

225g (8oz) Brussels sprouts, halved

225g (8oz) savoy cabbage, finely chopped

100g (3½ oz) cooked brown rice

1 large leek, finely chopped

2 tablespoons olive oil

1 tablespoon tamari sauce

SERVES 4

Method

Heat the oil in a wok or frying pan. Add the sprouts, leek and cabbage and cook for around 5 minutes or until softened. Add the brown rice and tamari sauce and warm it through. Serve and enjoy.

Cannellini Beans & Spinach

Ingredients

450g (1lb) spinach leaves
225g (8oz) cooked cannellini beans
4 tomatoes, chopped
3 tablespoons chives, chopped
2 cloves of garlic, crushed
1 large courgette (zucchini), chopped
3 tablespoons olive oil
1/2 teaspoon paprika

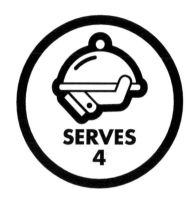

SERVES 4

Method

Heat the olive oil in a frying pan and add the courgette (zucchini), tomatoes, garlic and stir. Cook for 3 minutes. Add in the spinach, cannellini beans, chives and paprika and cook until the spinach has wilted and the beans are warmed through. Serve and enjoy.

Mixed Vegetable Casserole

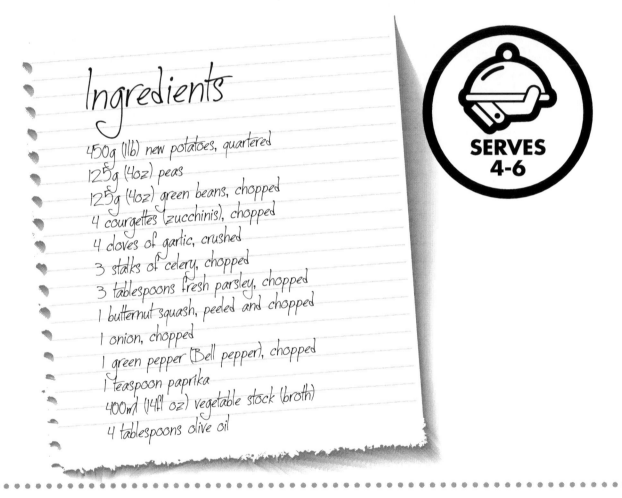

Ingredients

450g (1lb) new potatoes, quartered
125g (4oz) peas
125g (4oz) green beans, chopped
4 courgettes (zucchinis), chopped
4 cloves of garlic, crushed
3 stalks of celery, chopped
3 tablespoons fresh parsley, chopped
1 butternut squash, peeled and chopped
1 onion, chopped
1 green pepper (Bell pepper), chopped
1 teaspoon paprika
400ml (14fl oz) vegetable stock (broth)
4 tablespoons olive oil

SERVES 4-6

Method

Heat the oil in a frying pan and add the garlic, onion, potatoes and chopped butternut squash. Cook for 4 minutes. Transfer to a large casserole dish. Add to the casserole dish the courgettes (zucchinis), green beans, green pepper (Bell pepper), peas, celery and paprika. Pour in the vegetable stock (broth) and parsley. Bake in the oven at 190C/380F for 40 minutes. Serve with a little parsley.

Mixed Bean Pate

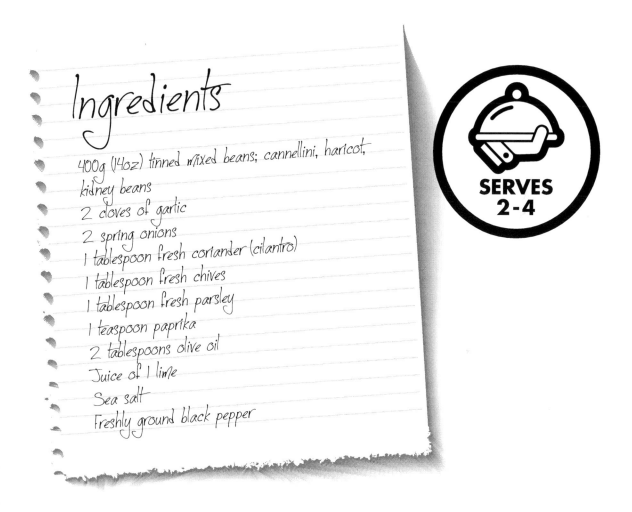

Ingredients

400g (14oz) tinned mixed beans; cannellini, haricot, kidney beans
2 cloves of garlic
2 spring onions
1 tablespoon fresh coriander (cilantro)
1 tablespoon fresh chives
1 tablespoon fresh parsley
1 teaspoon paprika
2 tablespoons olive oil
Juice of 1 lime
Sea salt
Freshly ground black pepper

SERVES 2-4

Method

Place all of the ingredients into a blender and process until the mixture becomes smooth. Season with salt and pepper and stir. Spoon the mixture into a bowl. Transfer it to the refrigerator and chill before serving.

Roast Autumn Vegetables

Ingredients

250g (9oz) peas, fresh or frozen
150g (5oz) button mushrooms
3 tablespoons toasted seed mix; sesame seeds, pumpkin seeds or flaxseeds
2 whole beetroot, unpeeled
2 cloves of garlic
1 butternut squash, peeled and cut into chunks
1 head of broccoli
2 tablespoons olive oil or ground nut oil
Sea salt
Freshly ground black pepper

SERVES 4

Method

Wash the beetroot then place it on a baking tray and sprinkle with salt. Place it in the oven at 200C/400F for around 1 hour or until tender. Place the squash on a separate baking tray and coat it with a little olive oil then transfer it to the oven and bake for around 45 minutes or until tender. In the meantime, steam the broccoli and peas for 5 minutes. Once the roast vegetables are cooked, heat the olive oil in a frying pan and add the garlic and mushrooms. Cook for around 3 minutes. Chop the beetroot into chunks and add it to the pan along with the butternut squash chunks. Sprinkle with seeds, season and serve.

Spicy Bean Burgers

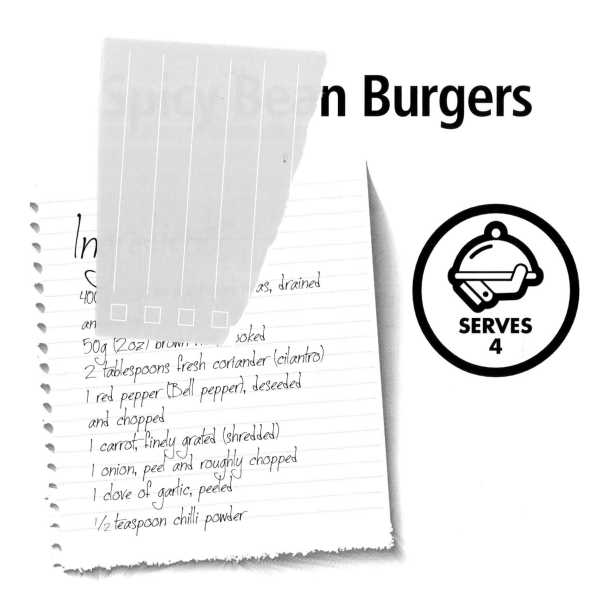

Ingredients

400g black-eyed peas, drained
and
50g (2oz) brown rice, soaked
2 tablespoons fresh coriander (cilantro)
1 red pepper (Bell pepper), deseeded
and chopped
1 carrot, finely grated (shredded)
1 onion, peel and roughly chopped
1 clove of garlic, peeled
1/2 teaspoon chilli powder

SERVES 4

Method

Place the black-eyed peas, carrot, garlic, onion, red pepper (Bell pepper), coriander (cilantro), chilli powder and brown rice into a food processor. Blend for a short time only, until the mixture is thick but not smooth. Scoop it out and place it in a bowl. Transfer to the fridge to chill for 20-30 minutes. Lightly grease a baking tray and preheat the oven to 200C/400F. Remove the mixture from the fridge and mould it into 8 patties. Bake for 20-25 minutes until golden brown. Serve with guacamole or tomato salsa and salad.

Vegetable Tagine

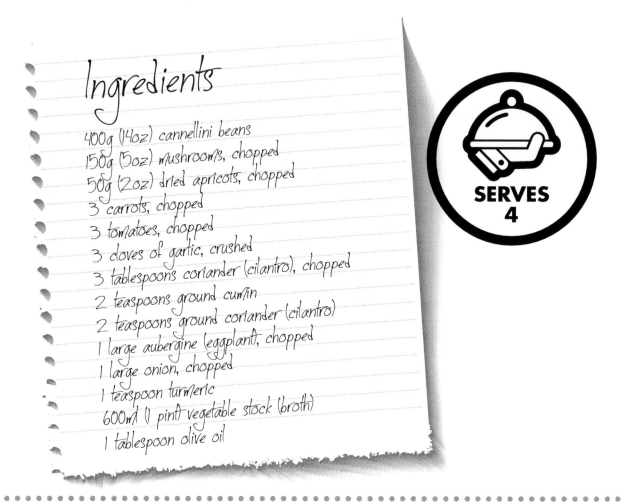

Ingredients

400g (14oz) cannellini beans
150g (5oz) mushrooms, chopped
50g (2oz) dried apricots, chopped
3 carrots, chopped
3 tomatoes, chopped
3 cloves of garlic, crushed
3 tablespoons coriander (cilantro), chopped
2 teaspoons ground cumin
2 teaspoons ground coriander (cilantro)
1 large aubergine (eggplant), chopped
1 large onion, chopped
1 teaspoon turmeric
600ml (1 pint) vegetable stock (broth)
1 tablespoon olive oil

SERVES 4

Method

Heat the olive oil in a large saucepan. Add the onion and garlic and cook for 4 minutes. Sprinkle in the spices and stir. Add the aubergine (eggplant), cannellini beans, tomatoes, carrots and mushrooms and cook for 5 minutes. Add the apricots. Pour in the vegetable stock, bring to the boil then reduce the heat and simmer for 10 minutes until the vegetables have softened. Stir in the coriander (cilantro).

Indian Style Stir-Fry

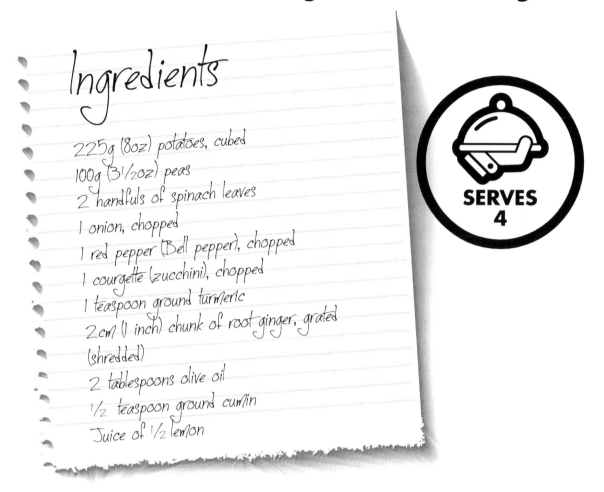

Ingredients

225g (8oz) potatoes, cubed
100g (3½oz) peas
2 handfuls of spinach leaves
1 onion, chopped
1 red pepper (Bell pepper), chopped
1 courgette (zucchini), chopped
1 teaspoon ground turmeric
2cm (1 inch) chunk of root ginger, grated
(shredded)
2 tablespoons olive oil
½ teaspoon ground cumin
Juice of ½ lemon

SERVES 4

Method

Heat the oil in a large frying pan or wok. Add the ginger, cumin and turmeric together with the onion and potatoes. Cook for 5 minutes. Add in the red pepper (Bell pepper), courgette (zucchini), spinach and lemon juice. Cook for 2 minutes. Add in the peas and warm them through. Serve with brown rice.

Caribbean Squash Casserole

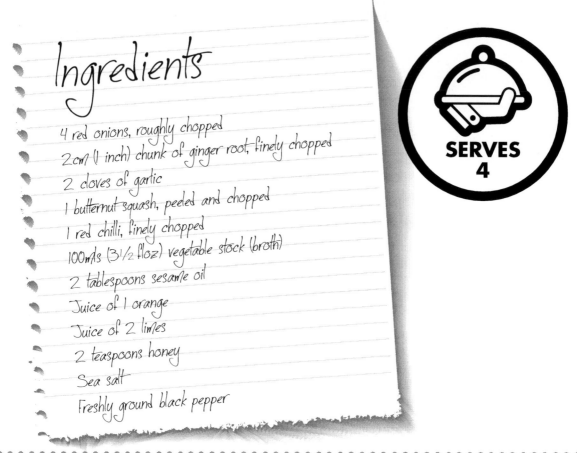

SERVES 4

Ingredients

4 red onions, roughly chopped

2cm (1 inch) chunk of ginger root, finely chopped

2 cloves of garlic

1 butternut squash, peeled and chopped

1 red chilli, finely chopped

100mls (3½ floz) vegetable stock (broth)

2 tablespoons sesame oil

Juice of 1 orange

Juice of 2 limes

2 teaspoons honey

Sea salt

Freshly ground black pepper

Method

Warm the sesame oil in a frying pan and add the onions, squash, garlic, ginger and honey. Cook for 3 minutes. Squeeze in the lime and orange juice. Pour in the stock (broth) and cook for 12-14 minutes until the squash is tender. Season with salt and pepper.

Braised Mixed Vegetables

Ingredients

SERVES 4

- 150g (5oz) baby corn
- 150g (5oz) mange tout (snow peas)
- 3 carrots, peeled and roughly chopped
- 2 large tomatoes, chopped
- ½ aubergine (eggplant), roughly chopped
- 2 tablespoons fresh chives, chopped
- 1 teaspoon smoked paprika
- 100mls (3½ floz) vegetable stock (broth)

Method

Place all of the vegetables, apart from the tomatoes, into a saucepan together with the stock (broth) and bring it to the boil. Reduce the heat, cover and simmer for 7-8 minutes or until the vegetables have softened. Add in the tomatoes and paprika. Stir until the tomatoes are warmed through. Sprinkle with chives and serve.

Hot Pot

Ingredients

400g (14oz) haricot beans
400g (14oz) black-eyed peas
400g (14oz) tomatoes, chopped
225g (8oz) mushrooms, sliced
150g (5oz) sweetcorn
2 onions, finely chopped
2 cloves of garlic, chopped
1 tablespoon paprika
1 red chilli, finely chopped
1 large handful of parsley
250ml (8fl oz) vegetable stock (broth)
1 tablespoon olive oil
1 tablespoon tamari sauce
Sea salt
Freshly ground black pepper

SERVES 4-6

Method

Heat the oil in a saucepan, add the garlic and onions and cook for 4 minutes. Add in the mushrooms, chilli, haricot beans, black-eyed peas, tomatoes, paprika and tamari sauce. Stir and cook for 5 minutes. Add in the stock (broth) and simmer for 15 minutes. Add the sweetcorn and parsley towards the end of cooking. Season with salt and pepper then serve and enjoy.

Chilli Stuffed Butternut Squash

Ingredients

- 450g (1lb) soya mince
- 400g (14oz) chopped tomatoes
- 200g (7oz) tin of kidney beans
- 2 butternut squashes, vertically cut in half, seeds removed
- 1 large onion, finely chopped
- 1 red pepper (Bell pepper), finely chopped
- ½ small courgette (zucchini), finely chopped
- 2 garlic cloves, crushed
- 1 teaspoon cayenne pepper
- 1 teaspoon cinnamon
- 1 teaspoon cumin
- ½ teaspoon chilli powder or more if you like it hotter
- 2 teaspoons tomato puree (paste)
- 1 tablespoon olive oil

SERVES 4

Method

Heat the olive oil in a saucepan, add the soya mince and cook it for 3 minutes. Add in the onion, red pepper (bell pepper), garlic and cook for 4 minutes. Add in the cayenne pepper, cumin, chilli powder, tomato puree (paste) and cinnamon and stir. Pour in the chopped tomatoes, courgette (zucchini) and kidney beans. Bring to the boil, reduce the heat and simmer for 15-20 minutes. Spoon the chilli into the hole in the squash. Cover with foil and transfer them to the oven. Bake on 200C/400F for 45 minutes, until the squash is soft. Remove the foil for the last 5 minutes.

Celeriac Cottage Pie

Ingredients

450g (1lb) soya mince
400g (14oz) chopped tomatoes
2 carrots, peeled and finely chopped
1 head of celeriac, peeled and chopped
1 leek, trimmed and finely chopped
1 large onion, chopped
1 tablespoon tamari sauce
1 tablespoon tomato puree
1 bay leaf
1 tablespoon olive oil
1 teaspoon fresh thyme, chopped
300ml (1/2 pint) vegetable stock (broth)

SERVES 4-6

Method

Heat the oil in a saucepan, add the mince and cook for 3 minutes. Add in the carrots and onion and cook for 8-10 minutes. Add in the tomatoes, tomato puree, tamari sauce, bay leaf, thyme and stock (broth). Bring to the boil, reduce the heat and simmer for 25-30 minutes. In the meantime boil the celeriac until it is soft and tender. Drain and mash it until smooth. Fry the leeks in a pan until they become soft. Combine the leeks with the mashed celeriac. Transfer the mince and vegetables to a casserole dish and top it off with the mashed celeriac. Place in the oven at 200C/400F for around 30 minutes until the top is slightly golden.

Lentil Bolognese

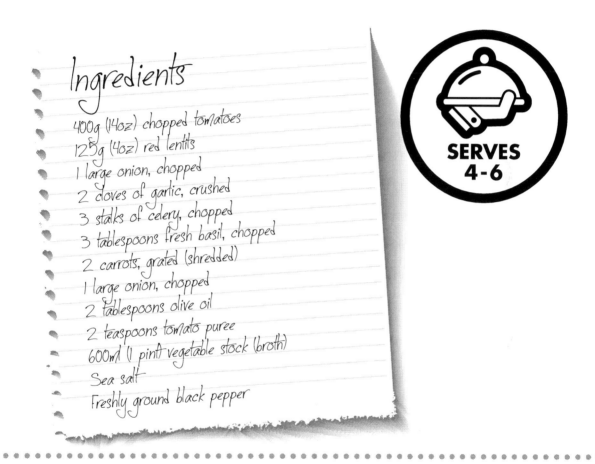

Ingredients

- 400g (14oz) chopped tomatoes
- 125g (4oz) red lentils
- 1 large onion, chopped
- 2 cloves of garlic, crushed
- 3 stalks of celery, chopped
- 3 tablespoons fresh basil, chopped
- 2 carrots, grated (shredded)
- 1 large onion, chopped
- 2 tablespoons olive oil
- 2 teaspoons tomato puree
- 600ml (1 pint) vegetable stock (broth)
- Sea salt
- Freshly ground black pepper

SERVES 4-6

Method

Heat the oil in a saucepan, add the garlic, onion, celery and carrot and cook until soft. Add the tomatoes, lentils, tomato puree, stock (broth) and basil. Cover and bring to the boil then reduce the heat and simmer for 15-20 minutes. Stir in the chopped basil. Season with salt and pepper and serve with vegetable 'spaghetti' (see recipe page 84) or baked potatoes.

Vegetable 'Spaghetti'

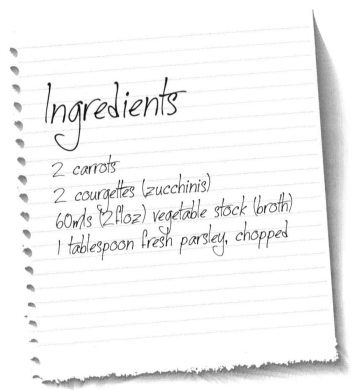

Ingredients

2 carrots
2 courgettes (zucchinis)
60mls (2 floz) vegetable stock (broth)
1 tablespoon fresh parsley, chopped

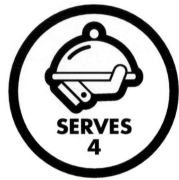

SERVES
4

Method

Peel the carrots and courgettes (zucchinis) into strips then slice them into 1cm (½ inch). Heat the stock (broth) in a saucepan, add the vegetables and boil them for around 3 minutes or until they are tender. Drain them, sprinkle with parsley and serve.

Mild Vegetable Curry

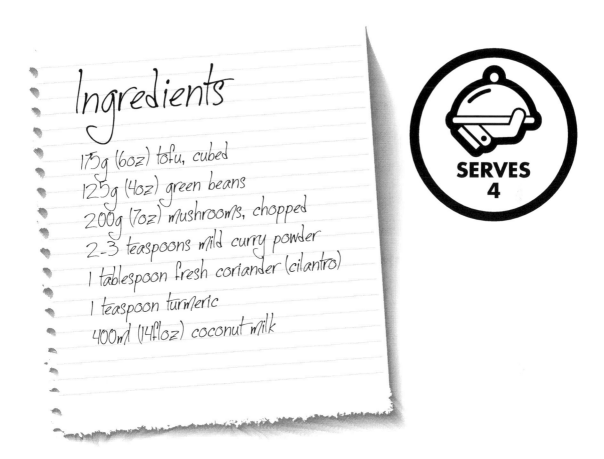

Ingredients

175g (6oz) tofu, cubed
125g (4oz) green beans
200g (7oz) mushrooms, chopped
2-3 teaspoons mild curry powder
1 tablespoon fresh coriander (cilantro)
1 teaspoon turmeric
400ml (14floz) coconut milk

SERVES 4

Method

Warm the coconut milk in a saucepan then add in the curry powder and turmeric and mix it well. Add the green beans, mushrooms, tofu and stir. Bring it to the boil, reduce the heat and simmer for 6-7 minutes until the vegetables are soft. Sprinkle with coriander (cilantro) and serve.

Thai Green Curry Vegetables

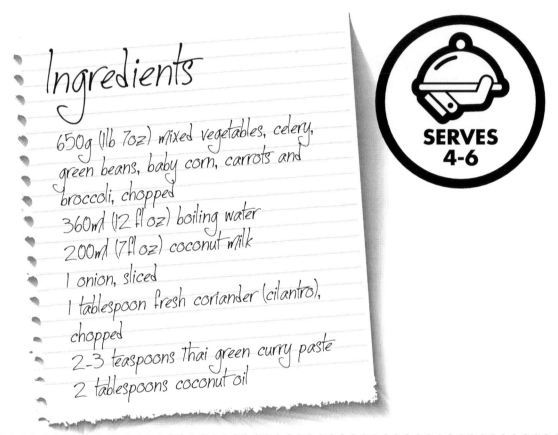

SERVES 4-6

Ingredients

650g (1lb 7oz) mixed vegetables, celery, green beans, baby corn, carrots and broccoli, chopped

360ml (12 fl oz) boiling water

200ml (7 fl oz) coconut milk

1 onion, sliced

1 tablespoon fresh coriander (cilantro), chopped

2-3 teaspoons thai green curry paste

2 tablespoons coconut oil

Method

Heat the coconut oil in a large pan. Add the onion and cook for 3-4 minutes. If you are using carrots, add them first and fry for 2 minutes. Add the remaining vegetables and cook for a further 2 minutes. Add the curry paste and the boiling water. Cover and simmer for 10 minutes until the vegetables are tender but firm. Stir in the coconut milk and add the coriander (cilantro). Heat through. Transfer to serving bowls and enjoy.

Fennel & Mushroom Casserole

SERVES 4

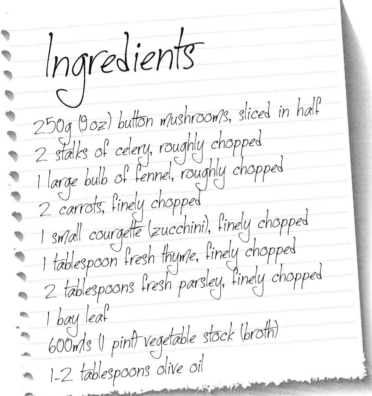

Ingredients

250g (9oz) button mushrooms, sliced in half

2 stalks of celery, roughly chopped

1 large bulb of fennel, roughly chopped

2 carrots, finely chopped

1 small courgette (zucchini), finely chopped

1 tablespoon fresh thyme, finely chopped

2 tablespoons fresh parsley, finely chopped

1 bay leaf

600mls (1 pint) vegetable stock (broth)

1-2 tablespoons olive oil

Method

Gently heat the olive oil in a saucepan and add the fennel, celery and carrots and cook for 5 minutes. Add in the mushrooms, courgette (zucchini), stock (broth) and bay leaf. Bring to the boil, reduce the heat and simmer for 15-20 minutes. Sprinkle in the herbs and stir. Serve and enjoy.

Quick Mushroom Stir-Fry

Ingredients

100g (3½ oz) brown rice or quinoa, pre-cooked
12 large mushrooms, finely sliced
1 red pepper (Bell pepper), finely sliced
1 green pepper (Bell pepper), finely sliced
1 bunch of spring onions (scallions) sliced diagonally
1 onion, finely sliced
1 large carrot, finely sliced
2 cloves of garlic, crushed
2 tablespoons sesame seeds
2 tablespoons sesame oil or olive oil
1-2 tablespoons tamari sauce
Sea salt
Freshly ground pepper

SERVES 4

Method

Heat the oil in a wok or frying pan and add in the onion, carrot and garlic. Cook for 2 minutes then add the rest of the vegetables and cook for around 3 minutes or until they begin to soften. Stir in the tamari sauce and add a splash of water if it starts to stick or is too dry. Stir in the rice or quinoa and warm it through. Season with salt and pepper and serve.

DESSERTS, TREATS & SNACKS

Strawberry Mousse

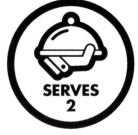

SERVES 2

Ingredients

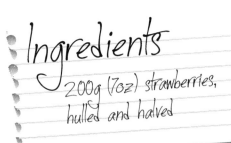

200g (7oz) strawberries, hulled and halved

125g (4oz) silken tofu
1 vanilla pod

Method

Place the strawberries in a small pan and simmer for 10-15 minutes or until they are completely soft. Set them aside to cool. Place the strawberries, tofu and vanilla into a blender and process until smooth. Spoon it into glasses or bowls and chill before serving.

Banana Ice Cream

SERVES 2-3

Ingredients

600mls (1 pint) full-fat coconut milk

2 ripe avocados
2 ripe bananas

Method

Place all the ingredients into a food processor or use a hand blender and blitz until smooth. Pour the mixture into an ice-cream maker and process according to the instructions for your model of machine. Serve straight away or freeze it. If you don't have an ice cream maker, place it in the freezer and occasionally whisk with a fork while it's freezing.

Fruit Kebabs
& Strawberry Dip

SERVES 4

Ingredients

400g (14oz) strawberries
150g (5oz) grapes
1 melon, cut into cubes

4 mint leaves
Juice of ½ lime

Method

Place 100g (3½ oz) of the strawberries together with the lime juice and mint leaves into a food processor and blitz until smooth. Thread the remaining grapes and strawberries onto the skewers. Serve along with the strawberry and mint dip.

Spiced Poached Peaches

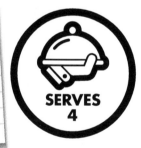

SERVES 4

Ingredients

4 large peaches
4 star anise
2 cinnamon sticks

300ml (½ pint) water
2 tablespoons honey

Method

Place the honey and water in a saucepan and bring to the boil. Add the peaches, star anise and cinnamon sticks. Reduce the heat and simmer gently for 10 minutes. Remove the peaches and set aside. Continue cooking the liquid for another 12-14 minutes until it begins to thicken. If necessary, return the peaches to the saucepan to warm them before serving.

Chocolate Muffins

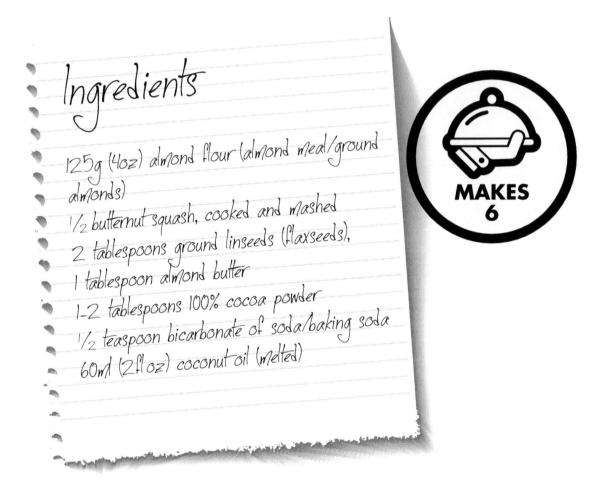

Ingredients

- 125g (4oz) almond flour (almond meal/ground almonds)
- 1/2 butternut squash, cooked and mashed
- 2 tablespoons ground linseeds (flaxseeds),
- 1 tablespoon almond butter
- 1-2 tablespoons 100% cocoa powder
- 1/2 teaspoon bicarbonate of soda/baking soda
- 60ml (2fl oz) coconut oil (melted)

MAKES 6

Method

In a bowl stir together the almond flour, flaxseeds (linseeds), bicarbonate of soda (baking soda) and cocoa powder. In a separate bowl, mix the squash, coconut oil and nut butter. Stir the squash mixture into the dry ingredients and mix well. Spoon the mixture into paper cases in a 6-hole muffin tin and transfer to the oven. Bake at 180C/350F for 30 minutes. Test with a skewer which will come out clean when they're cooked.

Strawberry & Mint Granita

SERVES 4

Ingredients

350g (12oz) strawberries   4 fresh mint leaves

Method

Place the strawberries and mint leaves into a food processor and blitz until smooth. Pour into a container and freeze. Every few hours beat the mixture with a fork. Freeze until firm and granular. Remove from the freezer 10 minutes before serving.

Apricot & Almond Truffles

SERVES 4

Ingredients

150g (5oz) almonds
150g (5oz) dried apricots
75g (3oz) raisins

2 tablespoons pumpkin seeds
1 tablespoon coconut oil
1 tablespoon warm water

Method

Place all the ingredients into a food processor and mix until chunky and sticky. Roll the mixture into small balls or alternatively press the mixture into the bottom of a loaf tin and cut into bars. These are a great handy snack for on-the-go.

Ginger & Lemon Tea

SERVES 1

Ingredients

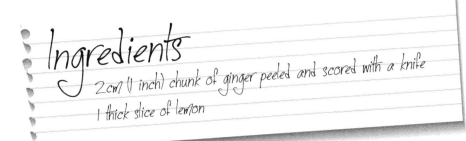

2cm (1 inch) chunk of ginger peeled and scored with a knife

1 thick slice of lemon

Method

Infuse the ingredients in hot water for 5 minutes before drinking.

Cinnamon Hot Chocolate

SERVES 1

Ingredients

300ml 1/2 pint almond milk

1/4 teaspoon cinnamon

1 1/2 teaspoons 100% cocoa powder

1 teaspoon honey, or to taste

Method

Place all the ingredients into a saucepan and mix well. Place on a medium heat and warm the milk. Remove it from the heat and whisk it really well to make it frothy. Pour into your favourite mug. Add a little extra cinnamon or honey if required.

Virgin Pina Colada

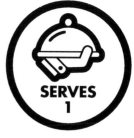

SERVES 1

Ingredients

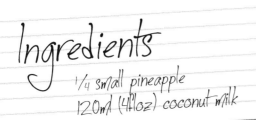

¼ small pineapple
120ml (4floz) coconut milk

Crushed ice

Method

Put all the ingredients into a blender or food processor and blitz until smooth.
Pour and enjoy.

Mango Milkshake

SERVES 1

Ingredients

120ml (4floz) almond milk or
coconut milk
½ ripe mango

Squeeze lime juice
Crushed ice

Method

Place the mango, almond/coconut milk into a blender with a squeeze of lime juice.
Blend until smooth. Stir in the crushed ice and pour into a glass.

Kale Chips

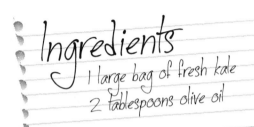

SERVES
4

Ingredients

1 large bag of fresh kale
2 tablespoons olive oil

Sea salt
Freshly ground black pepper

Method

Preheat the oven to 170C/325F. Remove the stalks from the kale and cut the leaves into bite-size squares, of around 4cms (2 inches). Put the oil, pepper and salt in a bowl and coat the kale leaves. Place them on a baking sheet, transfer them to the oven and bake for around 10 minutes or until crispy.

Baked Beetroot Chips

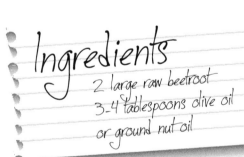

SERVES
4

Ingredients

2 large raw beetroot
3-4 tablespoons olive oil
or ground nut oil

Sea salt

Method

Preheat the oven to 200C/400F. Peel the beetroot and cut it into slices no more than 2-3mm thick (about the thickness of a coin). Put the oil, salt and pepper into a bowl and coat the beetroot slices. Lay the slices onto a greased baking tray. Transfer them to the oven and cook for around 10 minutes or until they are crisp.

Spiced Nuts

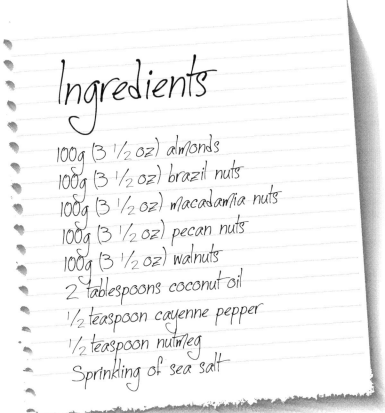

Ingredients

100g (3 ½ oz) almonds
100g (3 ½ oz) brazil nuts
100g (3 ½ oz) macadamia nuts
100g (3 ½ oz) pecan nuts
100g (3 ½ oz) walnuts
2 tablespoons coconut oil
½ teaspoon cayenne pepper
½ teaspoon nutmeg
Sprinkling of sea salt

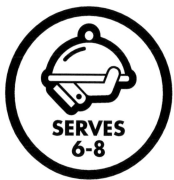

**SERVES
6-8**

Method

Heat the coconut oil in a large frying pan. Add the nuts, cayenne pepper, nutmeg and salt. Stir constantly for around 7-8 minutes. Store or serve as a snack. A variation is to substitute the nutmeg for curry powder.

Orange & Raspberry Fruity Water

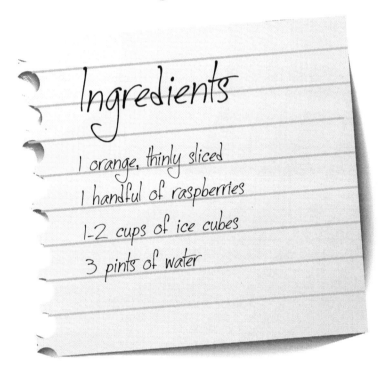

Ingredients

1 orange, thinly sliced

1 handful of raspberries

1-2 cups of ice cubes

3 pints of water

Method

A great replacement for fizzy, sugary drinks is fruit infused water. Fill a glass jug with water, add a small amount of fruit together with some ice and refrigerate it for 2-3 hours. You will only need a small amount of fruit, even less for stronger ingredients such a fennel and herbs. Experiment with some of these tasty combinations.

Cucumber & Fresh Mint
Pineapple & Mango
Apple, Ginger & Cinnamon
Kiwi & Lemon
Raspberry & Basil

Orange & Fennel
Apricot & Raspberry
Lemon & Ginger
Lime & Cucumber
Cucumber & Lemon

Strawberry & Lime
Orange & Thyme
Mango & Lime
Pineapple, Cherry & Lemon

CONDIMENTS

Avocado Salsa

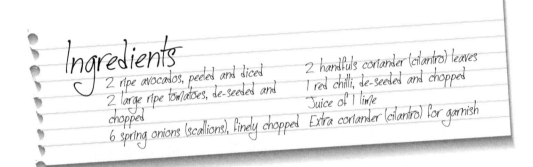

Ingredients

2 ripe avocados, peeled and diced
2 large ripe tomatoes, de-seeded and chopped
6 spring onions (scallions), finely chopped

2 handfuls coriander (cilantro) leaves
1 red chilli, de-seeded and chopped
Juice of 1 lime
Extra coriander (cilantro) for garnish

Method

Combine all the ingredients in a bowl and stir. Place in a serving bowl. Sprinkle with a little coriander (cilantro) to garnish. Serve with fish and meat dishes or even add to a salad.

Spicy Pineapple Salsa

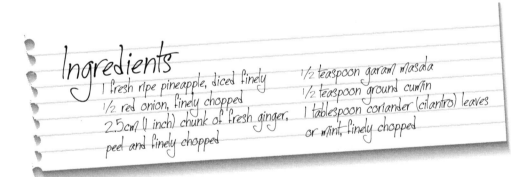

Ingredients

1 fresh ripe pineapple, diced finely
1/2 red onion, finely chopped
2.5cm (1 inch) chunk of fresh ginger, peel and finely chopped

1/2 teaspoon garam masala
1/2 teaspoon ground cumin
1 tablespoon coriander (cilantro) leaves or mint, finely chopped

Method

Place all the ingredients in a bowl and mix. Allow to sit and infuse for 20 minutes before serving.

Mint & Broad Bean Dip

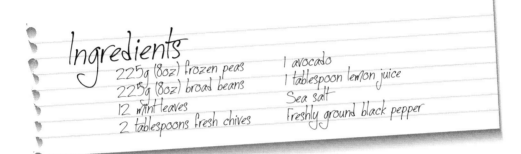

Ingredients

225g (8oz) frozen peas
225g (8oz) broad beans
12 mint leaves
2 tablespoons fresh chives

1 avocado
1 tablespoon lemon juice
Sea salt
Freshly ground black pepper

Method

Boil the peas in water until warmed through then drain them and allow them to cool.
Place all of the ingredients into a blender and process until smooth. Transfer the dip to
a bowl and chill before serving. It's delicious served as a dip for crudités.

Olive Tapenade

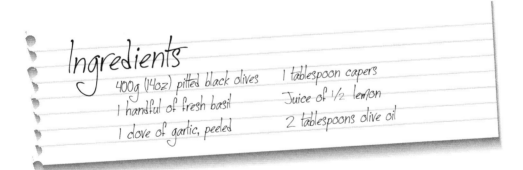

Ingredients

400g (14oz) pitted black olives
1 handful of fresh basil
1 clove of garlic, peeled

1 tablespoon capers
Juice of 1/2 lemon
2 tablespoons olive oil

Method

Place all the ingredients into a blender and process until slightly chunky.

Spinach Hummus

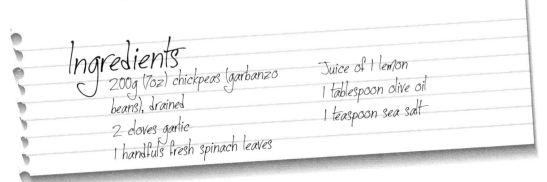

Ingredients

200g (7oz) chickpeas (garbanzo beans), drained
2 cloves garlic
1 handfuls fresh spinach leaves

Juice of 1 lemon
1 tablespoon olive oil
1 teaspoon sea salt

Method

Place all of the ingredients in a food processor and process until smooth. Serve as a dip or add a spoonful or two to salads.

Pomegranate Guacamole

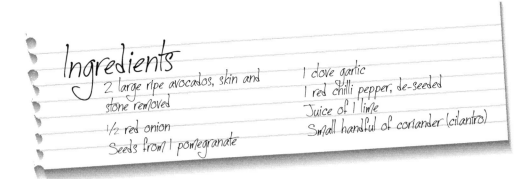

Ingredients

2 large ripe avocados, skin and stone removed
½ red onion
Seeds from 1 pomegranate

1 clove garlic
1 red chilli pepper, de-seeded
Juice of 1 lime
Small handful of coriander (cilantro)

Method

Place all of the ingredients, apart from the pomegranate seeds, into a food processor and blend until smooth. Season if required. Stir in the pomegranate seeds and sprinkle a few on top for garnish.

Lemon & Garlic Dressing

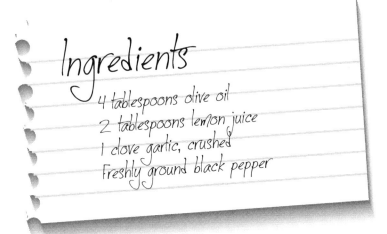

Ingredients

4 tablespoons olive oil
2 tablespoons lemon juice
1 clove garlic, crushed
Freshly ground black pepper

Method

Mix all the ingredients together and store or use straight away.

Orange & Cumin Dressing

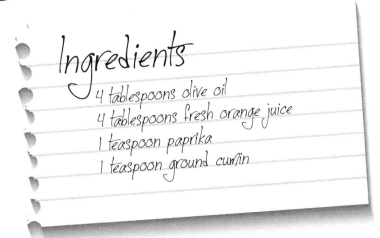

Ingredients

4 tablespoons olive oil
4 tablespoons fresh orange juice
1 teaspoon paprika
1 teaspoon ground cumin

Method

Combine all the ingredients in bowl and serve with salads. Eat straight away.

Printed in Great Britain
by Amazon